Living with PKU

A low protein life with Phenylketonuria

By Pauline O'Connor

"Completely fabulous. Brilliantly written."
Suzanne Ford, Metabolic Dietician & advisor to NSPKU.

"Absolutely brilliant & factual...lots of very good advice."
S.M., adult with PKU.

"Skilfully compiled...readable for anyone new to PKU."
C.H., new to PKU.

Living with PKU

A low protein life with Phenylketonuria

First published 2022

By Pauline O'Connor

© 2022 Pauline O'Connor

The right of Pauline O'Connor to be identified as author of this work has been asserted by her in accordance with s 77 and 78 of the Copyright, Designs, and Patents Act 1988.

All rights reserved. No part of this book may be reprinted or reproduced or utilised in any form or by any electronic, mechanical, or any other means, now known or hereafter invented, including photocopying and recording, or in any information storage or retrieval system, without permission in writing from the publisher.

Edition 1 (1.5)

ISBN: 978-1-7396356-0-2 (ebk)

ISBN: 978-1-7396356-1-9 (pbk)

Dedication

This book is dedicated to my family and friends, who work tirelessly to support my life with PKU.

Thank you all.

About the author

Pauline O'Connor was diagnosed at birth with Phenylketonuria (PKU), a rare inherited metabolic disorder. After a brain injury interrupted her career, Pauline turned to writing and uses her experience to help others with similar conditions. Alongside her work with patient organisations and charities, she publishes recipes and articles on www.pigpen.page

Also by Pauline O'Connor:

Living with Mild Brain Injury: *The Difficulties of Diagnosis and Recovery from Post-Concussion Syndrome.*

The Red Hat Stories. A fiction anthology.

Acknowledgements

I am grateful to those who helped ensure this book was completed, including:

My writing teacher for her continued critique, for sharing her extensive experience, and for her keen eye for a poorly-placed semi-colon. Here, have another one;

S.M. and Suzanne Ford for their enthusiasm, encouragement, and time;

The NSPKU for supporting me and other PKU families across decades;

Prof. Anne Green for her superb history detailing the development of the restricted diet treatment and of those pioneers who took a brave step into a nascent treatment;

My family and friends who endured the hours of procrastination and whinges involved in writing this book;

Finally, all the families, friends, health professionals, volunteers, and scientists, from across the years and around the world, who dedicate themselves to improving the lives of those born with PKU.

Contents

Introduction 15

Disclaimer 16
  A note about language & PKU   16

Part one: What is PKU? 17

1. What is PKU? 19
  Inherited Metabolic Disorders   20
  The mechanism of PKU   21
  Why are high phe levels in the blood a problem?   23
  Different types of PKU   24

2. How was PKU discovered? 27
  The mysterious green test result   28
  First publication and names   29
  PPA and phenylalanine   30

3. Pioneers of the first PKU Diet 33
  Why restricted diet?   34
  Removing phe from the diet   35
  An epic endeavour   37
  Sheila's fate   38

4. Diagnosing PKU today 39
  A closer look at blood phe levels   40

Blood phe levels used to diagnose PKU	41
Ideal PKU blood phe levels	42
My PKU diagnosis	44

5. Restricted diet therapy today 47

How much protein can someone with PKU have?	49
Protein and phe in food	50
Daily phe allowance and exchanges	51
Supplements	53
Diet for life	53

Part two: Why do we manage PKU?......................55

6. Why do we manage PKU?.................................57

The effects of being off PKU treatment	58
Returning to PKU treatment, it is never too late	60
Neurogenesis and Neuroplasticity	61

7. What causes the symptoms of PKU? 63

Phe toxicity	63
Competition at the blood/brain barrier	64
High blood phe and neurotransmitters	64
Serotonin	65
Dopamine	67
Eczema, skin repair, and Omega-3	69
Sleep and PKU	71

Part three: How do we manage PKU?....................73

8. Blood phe levels and testing 75
Why is blood phe testing critical? 75
Guthrie tests and blood spots 75
Blood phe monitoring at home 78

9. What else affects blood phe levels? 81
High blood phe levels 81
Low blood phe levels 84
Lessons from 40 years of blood spot levels 85

10. Making PKU clinics work for you. 87
Putting the patient first 88
Making effective use of your clinic 89
What if the clinic isn't working? 91
Food diaries 93

11. Supplements: a key battleground 95
Palatability of Supplement 95
Early PKU supplement 96
Maxamaid XP and Maxamum XP 98
Measuring older supplement doses 99

12. Supplements in the 21st century 101
Working out supplement dose 101
Supplement format 102
Supplement presentation and aesthetics 104
Glycomacropeptide, or GMP 107

Supplements in a nutshell 111

Remembering to take a supplement 112

13. Focus on food 115

Specialised PKU foods 115

PKU-friendly foods and food shopping 116

Aspartame in foods 118

Costs of PKU-friendly foods 119

14. Living with PKU, a personal story 121

Part four: PKU and mental health 127

15. Research on PKU and mental health 129

Current research into mental health and PKU 131

A need for support 133

16. Anxiety and PKU 135

Personal experience with anxiety 136

Mindfulness 137

Pause the anxiety treadmill 138

17. Social Isolation with PKU 141

Fad Diets & PKU 142

Eating out 144

Eating at home 145

Recipes and ideas 146

18. Abnormal food behaviours and PKU 147

Vomiting 148

Willingly eating non-PKU food	149
The avoidance of eating in public	151
When protein is the path of least resistance	153
19. PKU, depression, and fatigue	**155**
Fatigue	156
Acceptance is not resignation	157
20. Community and support	**159**
Benefits from the PKU community	162
How activity affects mood	163
21. Tell someone that you have PKU	**167**
Tips for talking to people about PKU	168
There is no shame in asking for help	169
Part five: Living with PKU	**171**
22. Planning with PKU	**173**
Habits and routine	173
Tips for a routine	178
23. PKU and being Hangry	**183**
Eat better, not more	184
24. Eating out with PKU	**187**
A little honesty about managing PKU in the real world	187
Example email	190
Tips when eating out spontaneously, or for low-key occasions 191	

25. Travel & emigrating with PKU 195

Sticking to the diet vs having a break   196

Longer trips   196

Dietician letters   197

Supplement while travelling   198

Eating and drinking while travelling   199

Emigrating with PKU   203

26. Celebrations with PKU 205

Cakes and birthday parties   207

Baking with PKU   209

PKU at Christmas   211

PKU adults and alcohol   214

27. Women and PKU 217

Pregnancy   217

Periods and PKU   219

28. Healthy eating and exercise with PKU 223

Healthy eating with PKU   224

Weight loss and PKU   225

PKU and exercise   227

Part six: Beyond restricted diet therapy 231

29. Other treatments in use globally 233

Large Neutral Amino Acid (LNAA) treatment   233

To sapropterin, and beyond   234

PEG-PAL, an injection for PKU	237
30. Living with PKU in the future	**241**
Gut absorption therapy in PKU	241
Other enzyme replacement therapies	242
Gene therapy	242
Reproducibility & safety	243
More research	244
Part seven: Resources	**247**
Units used	**247**
Abbreviations & Acronyms	**248**
PKU Support and Patient groups	**248**
Global Online Community	251
Possible financial support	**252**
Support for returning to treatment	**253**
Find a clinic	**254**
Support for pregnancy	**255**
Phe-free food lists	**256**
Treatment manufacturers	**257**
Other names for PKU	**259**
References	**260**
Bibliography	**270**
Glossary	**271**
Index	**276**

Introduction

I am not a health professional, nor an academic. Forty years of living with PKU means that I could be considered an expert through experience. However, while researching for this book, I came across aspects of the treatment of PKU which were new to me.

My approach to PKU and its treatments is continually developing. While I have tried to be objective and honest, my research is that of an amateur. I have included references throughout the text and in the bibliography. Please do use them, and remember that advances in research will soon outpace this book.

In fact, I hope this book will become obsolete. That it will one day be an interesting snippet of social history which documents how someone used to live with PKU, before advanced treatments consigned restricted diet therapy to medical history.

This book contains advice for meals, but it does not have recipes. These remain on my website because the phenylalanine (phe) analysis of foods, and recipes for commercial products, are continually updated, meaning a recipe's phe content will often change.

This book can be read from cover to cover, or you might prefer to dip into the different chapters. Please use the table of contents to guide you to a section of interest.

Disclaimer

This book should not be relied upon for medical treatment. Always speak to a health professional before making any changes to restricted diet therapies, or to any treatment plan.

A note about language & PKU

The language of older published papers regarding Phenylketonuria (PKU) can be uncomfortable to read, as they use 'mental retardation'. Now, we would avoid this by using the terms 'cognitive difficulties' or 'cognitive disabilities'.

There also used to be a classification of individuals with cognitive difficulties into categories, which include 'imbecile.' While these are difficult terms now, they were medical terminology at the time. This book avoids such phrases in favour of modern, and more sympathetic, terms.

PKU restricted diet therapy

For years, I said 'my diet' when explaining PKU or discussing the requirements of the condition. Now, everyone is on some form of diet; yet PKU stands apart. As a medically prescribed treatment, it more akin to diabetes than any of the above.

The restricted PKU diet is a prescribed medical therapy, where restricting food is a key part of the treatment. PKU is not a choice made because it helps one lose weight or 'just feel better, y'know'. It is not a fad or a choice, it is a medically regulated treatment. For this reason, I use the term 'PKU restricted diet therapy'.

I realise it is a bit of a mouthful, but then so is managing PKU.

Part one: What is PKU?

1. What is PKU?

I have been asked that question many times; by friends, colleagues, teachers, hospitality workers... I've even briefed medical staff on the ins & outs of PKU. There was a nurse sitting in at one of my clinics who wasn't aware of PKU. The consultant asked: 'Pauline, how would you describe PKU to my colleague?'

'I have Phenylketonuria, which is usually abbreviated to PKU.

PKU is an inherited metabolic disorder, with an incidence in the UK of approximately 1 in 10,000. Not all mutations result in fun super-powers, but dealing with PKU takes a heroic effort.

I inherited a mutated gene, which means my body cannot produce a particular enzyme which breaks down phenylalanine, one of the essential amino acids. Amino acids are the building blocks of protein, so I have to dramatically restrict the amount of protein I eat every day. If I eat too much protein, the amino acid which I can't process builds up in my blood like a toxin affecting my neurological and central nervous systems. Ultimately, too much protein in my food can lead to brain damage.'

At this point, most people say: 'What did you call it again?'

Occasionally, it is easier to start the explanation with: 'You know that warning on the back of soda cans "May contain Phenylalanine?" Well, it's me that they are warning.'

The next question is usually: 'Which foods have too much protein for you?'

'I can't eat meat, and yes, chicken and bacon are both meats. No fish, eggs, cheese, or dairy products. I can't have the vegetarian staples of Quorn, soya, and legumes like chickpeas, peas, & beans. They all have too much protein. I can eat most vegetables, but some of them, like potatoes, I can only have in restricted amounts.'

At some point, someone will again ask: 'Why you can't eat all that?'

'Because I'll get brain damage.'

'Yeah, but, like, why can't you save up and have a steak one night?'

'Nope, it doesn't work that way.'

Or when trying to find a restaurant we can all eat at. 'Can't you have one night off?'

'It doesn't work that way either.'

'Yeah, but...'

'I can't have a night off. It doesn't matter if it is your birthday or Christmas. If I eat too much protein, then this amino acid will build up in my blood and harm my brain.' For some reason, even though this isn't my fault, even though it is more difficult for me than for them, for some reason I will then say "sorry".

It is nobody's fault that we were dealt this hand. There was nothing our parents or grandparents did, or didn't do. It just is what it is. And it sucks. All we can do is make the best of it, and press for better treatments.

Inherited Metabolic Disorders

You may have noticed the phrase inherited metabolic disorder (IMD), above. There are hundreds of different IMDs, and most are caused by the reduced or missing activity of a single enzyme. PKU is one of the most common of these conditions, and it can be treated. Not all IMD's currently have a treatment.

In the US, and other countries, IMDs are called inborn errors of metabolism (IEM). For the rest of this book, I will use the term inherited metabolic disorder or IMD.

Frequency of PKU in the population

The incidence of PKU varies across different genetic makeups. A paper published in 2020 looked at the global incidence rate of PKU. The researchers found an average rate of 1 person with PKU in every 23,930 (1:23,930) births (Hillert, A et al., 2020).

However, the paper also found a marked variation in the incidence of PKU across different ethnicities. The number of people with PKU varies from as common as 1:4,500 births in Italy down to as rare as 1:125,000 for someone with Japanese ancestry. In Europe, which published PKU treatments guidelines in 2017, the incident rate which is accepted and used is 1:10,000. It is this rate which I will use in the book.

The mechanism of PKU

The food that you eat is broken down in the body. The main mechanism by which the amino acids in protein are broken down is by enzymes. Each amino acid has its own specialised enzyme which breaks the amino acid down into constituent parts. These parts are either used by the body in essential metabolic processes, or discarded in urine or faeces.

In PKU, the three organic compounds in the body of most interest are:

1. The 'PKU' amino acid: phenylalanine (phe)

This is an amino acid, which is one of the building blocks of protein in all the food which we eat. It is considered an essential amino acid as the human body does not make phe, so we need to eat it as part of our diet.

2. The enzyme: phenylalanine hydroxylase (PAH)

This is the enzyme which is produced by the human body to break down the amino acid phe. If PAH is impaired or missing, as in PKU, then phe is not broken down and remains in the blood stream. Over time, the phe in the blood stream can rise to dangerously high levels.

3. Another amino acid: tyrosine

When the enzyme PAH breaks down the amino acid phe, tyrosine is one of the products. This means that someone with PKU may not be able to make much tyrosine in their body. Tyrosine is also available in some foods. Sadly, these are mostly high-protein foods which are not suitable for the PKU restricted diet therapy. However, watercress is phe-free and has a relatively high level of tyrosine, as do okra and courgettes (SelfNutritionData, 2018).

This is the mechanism by which people with PKU end up with abnormally high levels of phe in their blood. They don't have enough of the enzyme PAH to break down the phe from the protein in their food. This phe which isn't broken down builds up in the blood, and the production of tyrosine in the body is impaired. High levels of phe in the blood can cause damage to the brain.

Why are high phe levels in the blood a problem?

As you know, a circulating blood supply is important for all the organs in our body, including the brain. The blood carries into the brain the oxygen, energy, and nutrients which it needs, and it takes away carbon dioxide and other waste products.

The brain is so essential that it is currently the only known organ of the body which has a protection mechanism, a security system if you like. This is known as the blood/brain barrier, and it is a network of tightly packed blood vessels. This network allows the entry of the essential items which the brain requires, e.g., glucose and oxygen. The blood/brain barrier also prevents harmful substances, like bacteria, from passing from the blood into the brain.

Because the amino acid phe is an essential nutrient, the blood/brain barrier doesn't recognise it as harmful and allows it to cross. This is fine if the blood arriving at the barrier has a normal level of phe. However, if the blood has a high level of phe, then more phe will cross the blood/brain barrier than the brain can handle. This is where the problems start.

PKU was identified due to the correlation between high levels of phe in the body, and severe cognitive impairments in the brain. Early in the discovery of PKU, researchers found that reducing the level of phe in someone with PKU reduces the level of cognitive disability. There is more on this in the chapter *How was PKU discovered?*.

However, this is not the only mechanism by which high levels of phe may cause damage. High levels of phe at the blood/brain barrier increases competition for other molecules which need to cross. This competition means that there are lower levels of some essential molecules crossing the blood/

brain barrier. There is more about the barrier in the chapter *What causes the symptoms of PKU?*.

Another mechanism though which high phe levels may cause damage is the disruption of signals in the brain. Neurons (brain cells) 'talk' to each other using signalling molecules called neurotransmitters. You may have heard of some of these, like serotonin or dopamine. High levels of phe in the brain may be able to disrupt some of these neurotransmitters (NPKUA, 2022). The signals the brain cells are sending out don't get to where they should be, which disrupts the normal function of the brain. You can find more on the specific effects of the disruption of serotonin and dopamine in the chapter *What causes the symptoms of PKU?*.

(As a side note, I received a separate brain injury from football. It led me to learn a great deal about the nature of brain damage, which I've written about in a previous book: *Living with Mild Brain Injury*.)

Different types of PKU

The amount of protein which people with PKU are allowed to eat will vary considerably from one individual to the next. This is because PKU is caused by an inherited mutation. Variance in the mutation means that everyone's PKU is a little different, and will have slightly different impairments to the PAH metabolism.

One research paper found more than 950 PAH gene variants (Blau, 2016). This huge number of variations means the amount of enzyme PAH which each person with PKU can make is different. In turn, this means each person can tolerate different amounts of phe in their diet. For more on the types of PKU, see *Diagnosing PKU today*.

Untreated PKU symptoms

This is a terrifying list for someone newly diagnosed, or who is currently not on a course of treatment. The key here is that these are the symptoms where someone with the most severe type of PKU is not treated, i.e., is eating a fully normal diet.

The most severe symptoms which may present in untreated PKU are:

- behavioural difficulties such as frequent tantrums;
- learning disabilities;
- eczema; perhaps a musty smell to the breath, skin, and urine;
- epilepsy, or jerking movements in arms and legs, or tremors;
- fairer skin, hair, and eyes than siblings without PKU. (Source: NHS, 2022)

Thank heavens for a treatment

PKU was not always treatable. In fact, PKU was only discovered within living memory. Sadly, the restricted diet treatment is difficult to stick to at all times meaning most of us will be familiar with some symptoms of high phe. But it is good to remind ourselves of them. We might be putting up with something not realising we can fix it!

Symptoms of high blood phe in treated PKU:

- anxiety, and/or depression;
- brain fog, slowed processing of information;
- difficulty with decision-making, problem-solving, and planning;

- difficulty controlling moods, particularly anger, irritability and frustration;
- inattention, problems with memory.

(These symptoms are sourced from personal experience and from others with PKU.)

As noted above, people with PKU traditionally have fairer hair and eyes than siblings. This has always led me to think of the 'dumb blonde' stereotype. Before treatment was available, people with severe PKU would have ailed rapidly.

Even those with mild PKU will have suffered continuous cognitive decline, and were likely to have had a lower IQ than average. Were people with untreated PKU the origin for the stereotype of the dumb blonde? Were they doomed to be the village idiot?

Fortunately, that is not the destiny for those with PKU today. This is thanks to the curiosity of a Norwegian chemist in the 1930s, and to a determined group of people in the 1950s, in Birmingham, UK.

2. How was PKU discovered?

As an inherited trait, PKU would have been a part of society for hundreds of years. However, it wasn't diagnosed until after the First World War. The discovery of PKU is due to the persistence of a mother, and the curiosity of a chemist.

Borgny Egeland gave birth to her first child, a girl, in Oslo in the late 1920s. Her daughter was initially healthy, but the child's development soon lagged considerably behind her peers. Borgny's doctor advised that her daughter's development would soon catch up, so the Egeland family waited.

Several months later, Borgny welcomed a second child. Her son was also born healthy, but soon exhibited the same intellectual disabilities as his sister. The boy's disability progressed at an increased rate, and Borgny was impelled to act. Along with intellectual impairments, the children shared a peculiar smell, difficulty walking, eczema, and fair hair.

By 1934, Borgny had visited many doctors and specialists for an answer as to why her healthy children had both become intellectually disabled. None had been able to diagnose her children, let alone treat them. She refused to accept this lack of explanation, and was convinced that there was a link between her children's disabilities and their other characteristics. While investigating the odd odour, her persistence led her to the door of Dr. Ivar Asbjørn Følling.

Dr Følling was both a chemist and physician. Whereas today, most doctors will have some knowledge of chemistry, this combination was rare at the time. Dr Følling also held a professorship in nutrient research at Oslo's University Hospital.

The mysterious green test result

Dr Følling was aware that problems with metabolism could lead to disabling conditions. But his first medical examination of the Egeland children did not offer any clues. Dr Følling then turned to chemical examination of the children's urine. At the time, diabetes was detected via the addition of ferric chloride to urine. A change in colour to purple or burgundy indicated a positive result for diabetes. Diabetes was not suspected here; nevertheless, Dr Følling conducted the test. The records aren't clear on why, perhaps he was going through a standard process of eliminating the knowns before investigating further. Whatever his thought processes, Dr Følling did find something.

The addition of the ferric chloride turned the urine of the Egeland children a deep green colour. It was not diabetes, but something was certainly odd. Dr Følling had never seen this reaction before, and he could find no similar reactions reported by colleagues or in research studies. After establishing that this was not simply a contaminated batch of urine, or caused by any of the medication, Dr Følling was able to conclude that the two children were producing something unusual in their urine.

At last, something was happening in Borgny Egeland's long search for answers. She carried litre upon litre of her children's urine to Dr Følling's lab as he doggedly tracked down the reason for this mysterious colour change. It took several months, but eventually phenylpyruvic acid (PPA) was identified. PPA is not supposed to be in human urine, so why was it there?

Extent of the problem

The chemist side of Dr Følling had identified the substance. Now, the physician side of Dr Følling took over to establish the extent of the condition. He tested 420 patients in local institutions, and found eight individuals with cognitive disabilities who also excreted PPA in their urine. This may not sound like many patients, but it is actually a very high rate. Eight in 420 equates to an incidence of roughly 190 in 10,000. In comparison, the current UK population has a PKU rate of 1 in 10,000.

Dr Følling noted that these patients also tended to have similar symptoms to Borgny Egeland's children: a peculiar musty smell, a fair complexion, difficulty walking, and eczema. He was collecting more data about the symptoms and incidence of his new-found condition.

These further investigations also suggested that this condition had a genetic link. Along with the original Egeland children, Dr Følling discovered several sets of siblings who shared the same problems. Moreover, some of these sets of siblings were from the same extended family, with closely related parents. This seemed too much of a coincidence, so Følling postulated that the condition must be hereditary.

First publication and names

Dr Følling published his initial findings in 1934, and gave this new condition the name Imbecillitas Phenylpyrouvica (Følling and Closs, 1938). This name would not be considered appropriate today, but it was chosen to reflect the main symptoms of the new condition; cognitive disability, and PPA in the urine.

Following the publication of Dr Følling's work, other medical professionals began to look for PPA in the urine of their patients with cognitive disability. As they found new cases, and wrote up their findings, they used various names for the condition. Along with Imbecillitas Phenylpyrouvica, the condition has also been called Oligophrenia Phenylpyruvica, and Følling's disease, in honour of the man who discovered it. I have not found any instance of a name which honoured the woman whose persistence sparked the whole discovery, Borgny Egeland.

This book will use Phenylketonuria, and the abbreviation of PKU. For information on other names for PKU, see *Other names for PKU* in the *Resources* section.

PPA and phenylalanine

Phenylpyruvic acid (PPA) had been identified in the urine, and gave this new condition its name. But how did it get there? There must have been an unusual mechanism in the metabolism of these patients which meant they produced PPA in their urine.

It was known at the time that PPA is a derivative compound of the amino acid known as phenylalanine (phe). For this reason, Dr Følling suggested that the PPA was excreted by the patients because they were unable to metabolise phe. Note: while I have found several papers which refer to this conclusion in Følling's original paper, I have not been able to find nor read the original paper to confirm.

Dr Følling theorised that an inability to process phenylalanine would mean that it accrued in the patient's blood to abnormally high levels before being broken down into PPA and excreted. We now know that his hypothesis was correct, but how did he prove it?

There was no test at the time which would allow Dr Følling to test the blood phe levels of patients. He decided to invent one. We have already seen that Dr Følling could think outside the box when he conducted a test for a condition which had already been ruled out. Now, he worked with a bacteriologist to find a strain of bacteria which could detect phe in the blood. Using this new diagnostic tool, Dr Følling was able to show that those patients who were excreting PPA in their urine, also had high levels of phe in their blood.

Dr Følling's early work established the existence of a new condition, its accompanying symptoms, and proffered a diagnostic tool. Following the publication of these initial findings, other professionals around the world began testing for, and finding, further incidences of PKU.

Dr Følling also continued to work on this new condition. He established that the genetic trait was recessive, and theorised on the possibility of detecting carriers. Sadly, despite all this work, there was still no treatment for PKU. Newly diagnosed patients had the comfort of a name for their impairment, but nothing more.

Borgny Egeland's children did not benefit from their pivotal role in the advancement of medical science. Sadly, the son died young, while the daughter lived into her forties in an institution. The world had to wait another twenty years for the development of a treatment.

3. Pioneers of the first PKU Diet

This will be a brief overview of how the dietary treatment for PKU was developed. The reason for this brevity is that there is a comprehensive account in Professor Anne Green's book, *Sheila*, which I highly recommend for those interested in the history of PKU.

This is another PKU story with several lucky coincidences, and it begins in Birmingham, UK, in the 1950s.

Impressing the boss

Twenty years after the discovery of PKU, and despite the development of a simple diagnostic test, screening for PKU was still not routine. At this time, a Dr. Horst Bickel started at the Birmingham Children's Hospital. His PhD had been in Aminoaciduria, or the study of unusual proportions of amino acid indicators in urine, and the chromatographic techniques required to measure them.

One morning, during the ward round, he asked his boss why the hospital was not testing for PKU. It proved a timely question, and a testing programme soon began. The team found a positive result on the third test. Given the rarity of the condition, this was an extremely lucky occurrence. How did that come about?

A mother's persistence

Mary Jones was, at the time, a mother of three in Birmingham. Her two older children were healthy and had developed normally. This experience with two healthy children meant Mary knew that something was impairing the development of her third child, Sheila. Concern led her to her local doctor, who in turn referred Sheila on to the Birmingham Children's hospital.

At the first examination, Sheila seemed to have some symptoms of this new condition. There was a bit of a delay, but eventually the hospital was able to test her urine and confirm that Sheila had PKU.

The team at Birmingham Children's Hospital were thrilled to have discovered a patient with this condition so quickly in their trial. Mary Jones was more interested in a treatment for her daughter, and simply would not accept that there was no therapy for this rare condition. It was her persistence which drove the doctors to develop a treatment for PKU.

Why restricted diet?

The understanding of the mechanism behind PKU was very limited at the time. Most of it was speculation rather than proven fact. For example, it wasn't known if the cognitive disabilities were caused by an excess of phe in the blood. They might have been caused by a deficiency of tyrosine, another essential amino acid which is produced when phe is metabolised. Alternately, the cognitive disabilities may not have been caused by the problems with phe metabolism. Could both the high phe levels and the disabilities be caused by another factor in the genetic inheritance? The team treating Sheila had to make their best guess.

A few years earlier, during his PhD, Dr Bickel had run a small trial to investigate the possibility that tyrosine deficiency caused the disabilities. The mechanism had not been proven, so the team turned to their other possibility; that the difficulties were caused by an excess of phe in the blood. With this as a working hypothesis, a logical step would be to assume that reducing or removing phe from Sheila's diet would improve her condition.

The two options available were to synthesise a completely phe-free food from scratch, or to remove phe from existing food items. The first option was prohibitively expensive, doubly so in a UK still undergoing food rationing following the Second World War. Thus, a restricted diet therapy became their focus. It is hard to escape the fact that the financial costs of a treatment has been a factor in PKU therapy right from the very beginning.

Removing phe from the diet

Adjusting the amino acid level in food was not entirely unprecedented. A method for removing phe from natural protein had been developed in the United States. This was achieved by first breaking a natural protein down into the constituent amino acids, and then filtering out the phe. However, this was the first time anyone had attempted to remove phe from food for the purposes of treating PKU. Fortunately, there was a source of expertise closer than the US; in London.

Dr Louis Woolfe

Dr Louis Woolfe worked at Great Ormond Street Hospital. He had experience in breaking down a milk protein into constituent amino acids to treat malnutrition. Dr Woolfe had already realised his technique may be useful in treating PKU, but had yet to find an opportunity to do so. When contacted by the team at Birmingham Children's Hospital, he shared his expertise with Dr Hickman and her team in the hospital laboratory.

Dr Evelyn Hickman

Dr Evelyn Hickman had established the Biochemistry laboratory at Birmingham Children's Hospital in 1923. Dr Hickman was a formidable lady who gained a scholarship to Birmingham University, and was one of only 27 women to study there in the 70 years before 1949. She gained a Bachelor degree in Chemistry, which was soon followed with a Masters. She then went to another university, where she formed an interest in dietetics, which she then lectured on at a third university.

Dr Hickman poured her knowledge and experience into setting up the Birmingham Children's Hospital laboratory in the inter-year wars. Alongside the demands of setting up and running the Biochemistry laboratory, she returned to Birmingham University and gained another Masters, this time in Biochemistry, and finally a PhD in Physiology. (I would dearly like to be the lazy kid on a group project with Dr Hickman.)

By 1951, when Mary Jones was pressing for a treatment for Sheila, Dr Hickman was running one of the few labs in the country capable of performing chromatographic diagnostic tests in a hospital environment. Her unique work, accompanied by a mostly female staff, held a critical role in both diagnosing Sheila, and in the development of a brand-new treatment.

The foul formula

The team filtered a protein derived from milk through activated charcoal to remove phe. This also removed several other essential amino acids from the formula, which then needed to be replaced. Through trials in the early treatment of Sheila, the team discovered that a completely phe-free diet was not a good treatment for PKU. Sheila's blood phe levels plummeted, and she soon swung from having far too much phe in her blood, to having far too little. The team discovered that Sheila needed a small amount of phe to prevent her body from breaking itself down (see *Catabolism* for more).

This was the discovery of something which everyone with PKU will now be familiar with. The need to keep our diet within that 'Goldilocks zone' of not too much phe, and not too little. Phe must also be ingested evenly across the week, and even across the day. We cannot simply save up all the phe allowance for a Friday night pub visit.

I have already shown how formidable Dr Hickman was in not allowing social norms, sexism, nor even two World Wars, prevent her from achieving her goals. She was no stranger to adversity, yet even she described the diet as both monotonous and distasteful (Green, 2020). Seventy years on, the formulas available for restricted diet therapy have evolved markedly. Yet, as I write this while trying to mask the taste of a lunchtime PKU supplement, that verdict brings a wry nod.

An epic endeavour

Despite the difficulties of adhering to the PKU diet, I do think of the persistent parents and the dedicated doctors & scientists who made a treatment possible.

- Borgny Egeland and Mary Jones who tirelessly sought help for their children.
- Dr Følling who agreed to help, and discovered a condition new to science.
- The coincidence of bringing a PKU child to a hospital where a new employee with experience in the field had recently set up a screening programme.

- That the hospital had a laboratory capable of conducting the accurate tests required for diagnosis and in developing treatments.
- The courage and persistence which Mary Jones had to stick with a treatment which would have unknown effects on her child.
- The skill and audacity of the doctors and scientists to delve into the unknown, and develop a new diet therapy in the midst of post-war rationing.

I am thankful that all these things came together to ensure that future generations of PKU children were not automatically consigned to poor IQ, dismissed as having bad brains, or dealt a life of institutions. I remain grateful, while hoping for more.

Sheila's fate

Sadly, adherence to the restricted diet caused significant difficulties for Sheila's family. Mary and her other children suffered due to the burden of the treatment. When Sheila was five, her diet deteriorated, and was eventually discontinued. The Jones family were forced to move, and lost contact with the team at Birmingham Children's Hospital Following her pivotal role, Sheila was lost to science for more than 30 years.

In 1987, an initiative which tested for PKU in mental health hospitals around Birmingham received a positive result for a 37-year-old woman named Sheila Jones. It was established that this was the same woman who had been so integral to advancing the understanding of PKU as a child. An attempt was made to return Sheila to the diet, but her cognitive disabilities were too great, and the attempt was abandoned.

4. Diagnosing PKU today

The experience of treating Sheila, and other adults with late-diagnosed PKU, demonstrated the importance of identifying PKU as early as possible.

Nappy test

In the 1950s, a test was developed which detected PKU by pressing a treated paper stick on to a urine-soaked nappy. This stick was coated with ferric chloride. If the baby had PKU, the PPA in the urine on the nappy would turn the stick green. This was a simple and quick test which became known as 'the nappy test'.

The nappy test was rolled out across the UK. Though patchy at first, the development of a nationwide screening programme marked a turning point in understanding the extent of PKU in the population. Though the condition was still rare, the early diagnosis meant that the brains, and lives, of those with PKU could be protected from birth.

The screening programme was such a success that most newborns in England and Wales were tested for PKU by the late 1960s. The speed meant that within two decades, PKU progressed from an untreatable degenerative condition, through the development of a dietary treatment, and on to a mass programme of newborn screening.

Guthrie cards and blood spot tests

The mass use of the 'nappy test' revealed that it was not as reliable as hoped. There were too many patients producing a false negative. Fortunately, a new diagnostic method was developed in the US by Dr. Robert Guthrie. The test involved spotting blood onto an absorbent card. Once the blood dries, a sample of the card with the dried blood is removed for testing. This test is still in use, and will be familiar to PKU families around the world as the 'Guthrie test', or the 'blood spot test.'

A closer look at blood phe levels

Blood phe levels are used to diagnose PKU. If they are too high in a person on a normal diet, then that person is likely to have PKU. Blood phe levels are also used to discover how much natural phe in the diet someone with PKU can tolerate, i.e., to work out someone's daily phe allowance. For more on phe allowance and exchanges, see *Restricted diet therapy today*. Blood phe levels are also used on a daily, weekly, or monthly basis by healthcare professionals and families to monitor potential damage to the brain.

Basically, blood phe levels are important. So let's start to put some numbers on them.

Blood phe in the UK, New Zealand and several other countries, are measured in micro-moles per litre. This will often be written as µmol/L. This is a standard measure which will be familiar to chemists. In other countries, including the US, blood phe levels are reported in mg/dL. As an example: the range 120-360 µmol/L may also be expressed as 1.35-4 mg/dL.

Do not be alarmed if you are not familiar with these units. Just as everyone is different, so are blood phe levels in people both with and without PKU. What we need to know for monitoring or diagnosing PKU is whether the blood phe levels sit within an acceptable range.

PKU is a form of Hyperphenylalaninemia

Hyperphenylalaninemia (HPA) is the name given to the condition of having too much phe in the blood. It typically refers to someone whose PAH enzyme isn't functioning as it should. HPA could conceivably happen if someone decided to dose themselves up on phe to a point that their body isn't able to cope. Normally, HPA is caused by an Inherited Metabolic Disorder (IMD).

Blood phe levels used to diagnose PKU

Blood phe level in someone without PKU

This is sometimes called the 'normal' range. Being called abnormal is something which follows someone with PKU around; it can have an impact on mental health. So, I prefer to say that someone without PKU and eating an unrestricted diet would have a blood phe level below 120µmol/L (below 1.35mg/dL) (Medscape, 2017).

The following blood phe level ranges are from the 'NHS evidence review: Sapropterin for phenylketonuria' published in 2018. Remember that these blood phe ranges used to diagnose PKU refer to phe levels when the PKU is not treated.

Classical PKU

The NHS review reported that someone with an untreated blood phe level over 1200µmol/L is considered to have classical PKU. This refers to the most severe form of PKU, as it was initially diagnosed. People with classic PKU usually have a low phe allowance. I have classic PKU and am allowed 5 phe per day.

Mild PKU

If someone has untreated blood phe levels between 600 and 1200μmol/L, they are considered to have mild PKU. This means that, while they still cannot eat a normal diet, they have more active enzyme in their body so can metabolise, and therefore safely eat, more phe in their diet.

Mild Hyperphenylalaninemia

Someone with untreated blood phe levels above the normal range of 120μmol/L, but below 600μmol/L, has mild hyperphenylalaninemia. Wow, that is a mouth full! It is frequently shorted to mild HPA.

Remember, these are untreated levels

It is important to remember that these are untreated blood phe levels; i.e, where someone is not restricting their diet. I first read about these diagnostic ranges as a child. It was just after a particularly good blood phe level. 'Hey mum! I don't have PKU! I can eat normally. Look, my last blood spot was under 120, so I don't have it!'

There followed a difficult conversation about untreated PKU vs treated, and that my blood test was taken while I was on treatment. And how PKU is not yet curable. And that, although I had been particularly good on my diet that month, there would still be a different pot on the dinner table for me every night.

Ideal PKU blood phe levels

As with many things, little in PKU is simple. The blood phe level guidelines differ across the globe. My greatest hope for PKU blood phe monitoring is that a kit allowing us to measure our phe levels at home will be available in future. This would allow us to monitor our blood phe and adjust daily. My second great hope is that PKU clinicians and researchers worldwide will eventually agree on safe blood phe levels.

The current standards, at the time of publication, are:

UK and European guidelines

- Children under 12-years old: 120–360 µmol/L
- Pregnant women, including those attempting to conceive and who are breast-feeding: 120–360 µmol/L
- Children over 12-years-old, and non-maternal adults: 120–600 µmol/L

These were agreed in 2017 (van Spronsen, et al., 2017).

US guidelines

120-360 µmol/L (1.35-4 mg/dL) in patients of all ages for life.

These guidelines were released in 2014 (NPKUA, 2014).

Australia and NZ

Children up to the age of 12: 120-360µmol/L.

It is important to note that the Australian guidelines (Inwood, A et al., 2021) suggested that over 12 years of age, the patient may decide to accept phenylalanine levels above 360µmol/L. The implication being that patient should be aware that levels over this constituted harm.

The same source also noted that research into subtle neurocognitive changes, such as depression and anxiety, is inconsistent in adult patients with phe levels between 360 & 600µmol/L. This range is within the wider range of blood phe levels accepted in the UK and most of Europe. The Australian guidelines, dating to 2016, go on to call for more research into these possible problems. I would be very keen to see some too.

My PKU diagnosis

By the time I was born in Scotland at the start of the 1980s, newborn screening was well established. However, there was still the need to wait a few days for the phe to build up in the blood. I was diagnosed with classic PKU at 6-days old, and immediately started on a restricted diet therapy.

My diagnosis was a shock, as it is to any new parent. However, a diagnosis and treatment is a remarkable achievement for an inherited metabolic disease which was discovered less than 50 years earlier. Despite the shock, this was good news. Of all the people born with PKU in the history of the mutation, I had been born in the minuscule window of time when we have had both:

- the tools to diagnose PKU early, and
- the knowledge to treat it before severe damage can occur.

When you stop and think about it, this is an incredible piece of good luck.

There was more luck to come. My parents tell me that there was a centralisation of PKU in Scotland at the time of my birth. Though I was diagnosed in a small hospital in between the two cities of Glasgow and Edinburgh, I was admitted to Royal Hospital for Sick Children in Glasgow for confirmation. It was there that I came under the care of Professor Forrester Cockburn.

Professor Cockburn had studied phe for decades. His thesis, presented in 1966, was on 'Phenylalanine — its role in infant nutrition and disease.' In the following decades he continued to work in the field, and by the time I came under his care he held the Chair (professorship) of Child Health at the University of Glasgow.

Decades of experience in metabolic disorders, and a dedication to child health, had led Dr Cockburn to live on the PKU supplement to prove that it worked. Fortunately for me, he also remained a clinical professor and continued to work in hospitals. My treatment began in the best care possible, and my parents were able to access expert support. This was to prove invaluable when we moved to the other side of the world, and encountered more patchy care.

Initial phe challenges showed that I had classical PKU, and could only tolerate 200 mg of phe in my diet every day. This amounts to 4 phe, or 4 grams of protein. My mother had to stop breastfeeding immediately, and instead began the challenge of feeding a bitter amino acid formula to her newborn.

The clinical team at the University of Glasgow also had a dietetics department. My parents had 24 hour access to the dieticians for any help. My mother recently gave me the decades-old notebook containing my first diet, which makes for scattered reading as the challenges of toddlers intervened with attempts to write things down.

I also have two siblings, and neither of them has PKU. But that doesn't mean they weren't affected by it. They grew up on the PKU biscuits, in case any non-PKU treats were left where I might find them. When, in our thirties, a type of PKU wafer biscuit was discontinued, my brother also mourned the loss.

5. Restricted diet therapy today

The "red list" of foods which many with severe PKU can't eat:

- Meat: all types of meat. Yes, chicken is meat!
- Fish: all types, including shellfish.
- Eggs: again, all types; chicken, duck, quail… even liquid pasteurised egg.
- Cheese: all types of cheese which are high in protein. Some new vegan cheeses are allowed, but not all vegan cheese. It depends on the main ingredient and how much protein is added during processing.
- Most nuts and seeds: This is one of the main ways in which the PKU therapy differs from a vegan diet. Nuts and seeds are everywhere in the vegan diet. A vegan may easily boost their protein intake by adding mixed nuts to a breakfast bowl, or pumpkin seeds to breads, or using chia seeds to replace egg in baked foods.
- Many baked foods such as bread, cakes, & biscuits are not allowed. Yep, no picking up a birthday cake from the local bakery, or grabbing a quick panini as a working lunch. (This is probably my biggest problem area. I have a sweet tooth, and cakes are just everywhere.)
- Soya & Tofu: This is another key difference between the PKU therapy and a vegan or vegetarian diet. Soya beans, like most legumes, are high in protein. All beans and most legumes are a seed, a package formed by evolution which contains everything a tiny seedling will need to germinate. This includes a fairly high level of protein. Tofu, or soya bean curd, is made by soaking soya beans before grinding them into a milk-like substance. The curds of this soya liquid

- are then condensed into a block, tofu, which is very high in protein.
- Quorn: Most Quorn is made from a fungus. Before you say 'ewww', mushrooms are a fungus. Someone with PKU can eat mushrooms freely, but the fungus in Quorn is different and is fermented during production. It is also often bound using egg, which adds more protein into the product.
- Aspartame, an artificial sweetener: aspartame contains a very high level of phe, and thus is dangerous for people with PKU. Sadly, it can be found in everything from sodas to medicines. Common brand names for aspartame include NutraSweet, Equal, or Canderel. Someone with PKU must carefully check the ingredients of all food, drinks, and medicines to be certain it doesn't contain aspartame. It may be labelled as simply additive 'E951'. All products with aspartame will be labelled, but it is hard to explain to a bar tender at 11pm why you need to check the ingredients list for your drink.

So, what do we actually eat? The restricted diet therapy for my classic PKU allows most, but not all, fruits and vegetables. There are medically synthesised pastas and rice substitutes for people with PKU. There is also a medical flour, so I bake my bread, biscuits, & etc. To supplement this diet, I need to take prescribed supplements every day which ensure I have the correct intake of nutrients like iron and calcium. And that, in a nut-shell, is the PKU diet.

Except that it isn't. As the Birmingham Children's hospital team found when they were developing the first therapy for PKU, every diet must have some phe in it.

How much protein can someone with PKU have?

To work out how much phe someone with PKU is allowed per day, they must take a challenge trial. In this trial, the metabolism is challenged by eating a bit more phe and seeing what happens to the blood levels. That is currently the best science can do.

On average, someone with PKU is usually allowed less than 500 mg of phe per day (MacDonald et al., 2020). Do note that this is an average across many people with PKU. Your clinic or health professional will advise how much phe you are allowed.

The genetic variation behind the mechanisms of PKU leads to a massive variance in the amount of phe which a person may be able to eat. Some people with PKU can only tolerate low levels of phe in their diet. Others may be allowed enough phe daily to eat a MacDonald's burger.

Furthermore, the amount of phe a person can tolerate may change throughout their life-time. This is especially true for a woman with PKU who would like to have a child. Child bearing with PKU becomes a carefully controlled process, in which PKU specialists closely monitor the protein requirements of the mother and the growing baby. These needs must be fully met, without endangering either baby or mother.

It is definitely possible for someone with PKU to safely carry a pregnancy and to have a healthy child. Specialist help and support is crucial at this critical time, and there is a little more on this subject in the chapter *Women and PKU*.

Variations in phe allowance

As I said above, phe tolerance varies from one person with PKU to another. But, that doesn't stop the 'how much phe are you on?' question being the first one asked whenever those with PKU meet. The curiosity is understandable. People with PKU meet so rarely that any chance to discuss the diet with someone who understands the challenges is welcome.

There is always a tinge of envy and pity in these conversations. To someone who does not have to think about it every day, there doesn't sound like much of a difference between an allowance of 4 phe and an allowance of 8. But, being able to have an extra phe with a meal might mean you can buy lunch, rather than needing to prepare something in advance. Any extra phe allowance can make a huge difference.

And it isn't a matter of simply avoiding the ham in a sandwich, the bread itself contains protein. As an example, I am allowed 5 phe, or 5g of natural protein, per day. That is the protein equivalent of one slice of wholemeal bread. If I had a single slice of bread for lunch, everything else I eat that day must be phe-free. A massive ask!

Protein and phe in food

Protein in food is a mixture of various amino acids grouped together. My apologies to any nutritionists and chemists, but I find the easiest way to explain the relationship between protein and phe is with a simple analogy. I like to think of amino acids as being the building blocks of protein. The amino acid of concern in PKU, phenylalanine (phe), is only one of these building blocks. However, removing a single amino acid from all the protein in a food item is difficult. Furthermore, not all foods have the same proportion of amino acids in the make-up of their protein.

I'll use a food-cupboard staple as an example. Tinned tomatoes usually come with a nutritional information label on the side of the can. This will typically state that the tomatoes contain about 1g of protein per 100 grams. But, the proportion of phe in the protein of tomatoes is actually relatively low. Or to put it another way, fewer blocks of phe are used when building the protein in a tomato. So, someone with PKU would be allowed to eat more tomato than that '1g of protein' might suggest.

What does "phe-free food" mean?

If all food has protein, how can any food item be considered phe-free? In the UK & Europe, A food item which has 0.5g of protein per 100g, or less, is considered to be a phe-free food. These are commonly referred to by those with PKU as 'free foods'. This is our holy grail, a food which we can eat without needing to measure or count.

Examples of phe-free foods include: apples, sweet potato (but not regular potato!), herbs & spices, and honey. Not all fruits and vegetables are considered to be phe-free. There are links to phe-free food lists in the *Resources* section.

You are starting to see the complications here. How does someone with PKU manage to remember the exact phe content of each type of food, whether it is phe-free or not, and how much of that food they are allowed to eat? This is where the idea of a daily phe allowance comes in. This allowance is commonly known as exchanges, or some may call them protein points. I will use the terms exchanges or daily phe.

Daily phe allowance and exchanges

An exchange refers to 'a measured quantity of food that can be exchanged or substituted for another food of equivalent phenylalanine content' (MacDonald, 2021). Someone with

PKU will be given a certain number of exchanges, which is the total amount of protein they are allowed to eat in a single day.

A general rule of thumb holds that one gram of protein contains 50 mg of phe. As foods are tested for their phe levels, there are a few exceptions where that proportion is significantly different. (As in the example of tomatoes given above.) However, the generally accepted rule of thumb is: 1g of protein contains 50mg of phe.

In the UK, this is also what dieticians and people with PKU commonly refer to as an exchange. So, 1g protein = 50mg phe = 1 UK exchange.

I wish there was a universal system across the world which set a standard for the amount of phe in each exchange. But there simply isn't.

Exchanges are different in the US, where one exchange is 15mg of phe. This means in the US 1g protein = 50mg phe = 3.5 US exchanges (NPKUA, 2011)

For the avoidance of doubt, and unless otherwise stated, all references to phe or exchanges in this book refer to the UK system.

What does one phe look like on a plate? One phe might be 80g of boiled potatoes, which contains 1g of protein. Or, 160g of a low-phe coconut yoghurt. Or 7g of pine nuts.

Each of these foods might be a meal, or a part of a meal, and is counted towards the total phe allowance which that person's phe tolerance allows them to eat in a single day. These examples show how much a person with PKU must juggle their diet to eat enough food to survive, while still staying within their phe tolerance.

Supplements

Along with ensuring that we only eat a prescribed amount of phe, someone with PKU also must take supplements. I grew up calling these a medicine or a special drink, but supplement is the best word. This is because the supplement provides the body with all the essentials which it still requires, but which we can't get from the small amount of allowed food.

The PKU restricted diet therapy controls the amount of protein to limit the amount of phe ingested. But phe is only one of the essential amino acids which make up protein. Because these essential amino acids are all mixed in food, the diet therapy doesn't just restrict the amount of phe, it restricts all these other amino acids too.

The body still needs these amino acids, just as it needs all the other vitamins and minerals which are removed by the restricted diet therapy. This means things like calcium because we can't have milk or dairy products. Or iron because we can't eat meat. Omega three fatty acids are plentiful in fish, but those with severe PKU can't eat fish.

This is where the supplement comes in. It provides all the other essential things which are restricted on the PKU diet therapy. There are many types of supplements, and they come in different formats, like ready-made drinks or tablets. There are two chapters on supplements in the section called *How do we manage PKU?*. For now, just remember that they are an essential part of the restricted diet therapy.

Diet for life

It was once practice in the UK to remove children from the PKU restricted diet therapy at the age of 8. Then, it became common to do so after the teenage years. The reasoning behind these decisions was the belief that the brain was fully developed by that point; therefore high levels of phe crossing the blood/brain barrier was no longer of concern and could no longer cause damage.

Thanks to research in neurogenesis and neuroplasticity, we now know that the brain continues to grow and make new connections throughout a person's lifespan. I have explained more about neurogenesis and neuroplasticity in *Why do we manage PKU?*. When this new research is applied to PKU, we can see that there is no safe time to permit high phe levels, nor the disruption and damage which they cause.

This is why 'diet for life' became the norm for PKU treatment around the world. Indeed, it was in 1993 that 'diet for life' became standard in the UK. This is slowly changing into 'treatment for life' as new therapies, beyond restricted diet therapy, are developed. (There is more on these new therapies in the section *Beyond the restricted diet therapy*.) This late change means that there are people who were diagnosed with PKU, and initially treated, who are now no longer being treated for their PKU.

Three keys to PKU restricted diet therapy

To recap, someone with PKU needs to focus on three things:

- Not eating approximately 85% of foods which are too high in protein.
- Eating enough of the remaining foods to meet their personal phe allowance.
- Taking enough supplement to ensure their body isn't missing anything.

The average person with PKU usually ends up with a more advanced knowledge of nutrition & metabolism than the average person without PKU. It is this knowledge which helps us understand why we must manage our PKU.

Part two: Why do we manage PKU?

6. Why do we manage PKU?

It is a good question. Why stick to the diet? Why all the measuring? And the label reading, and the blood spots, and the anxiety, and the guilt! Why?

Brains.

You may have heard this from parents, dieticians, doctors, teachers, (possibly even from zombies) but it really is all about the brains. People living with PKU are the most qualified when it comes to living with PKU and I can confirm: Yes, it is all about the brain. Not just IQ wise, but in how we feel and what we do.

It is not my intention to scare, lecture, or condemn. Managing PKU, whether by restricted diet therapy, or the newer treatments, is no easy task. It is a group effort which needs support and the willpower to pick yourself up, time and again. This effort is worthwhile, it means we avoid hurting our brains.

There is no other organ which is so uniquely you. The brain contains an enormous amount of information. It is the instruction manual for running the body. The brain helps you decide how to react to other people. The brain is integral to how you interpret the world around you, and how you wish to interact with that world. Your brain is you, and you are your brain. We need to care for our brains.

It is nobody's fault that we were dealt this hand. There was nothing our parents, or grandparents, did. It just is what it is, and it sucks. We are left to make the best of it.

Damage from PKU is brain damage

As I said, I do not intend to scaremonger, only to emphasise the seriousness of PKU. At the age of 34 I suffered a brain injury during an amateur football match. It was initially diagnosed as concussion. But, after 15 months and numerous brain scans, the neurologists were able to find the bleed in the back of my brain.

During my recovery, keeping my PKU under control was a key focus. I wanted to avoid having to manage high blood phe levels and a brain injury at the same time. My blood phe levels stayed within the European guidelines while I followed the regimes of physiotherapy and medications. However, I found that many of the symptoms of my diagnosed brain damage were the same as those I had previously experienced with high phe levels. These included:

- headaches, and migraines;
- lack of co-ordination, and tremors;
- brain fog, and reduced executive function;
- high levels of anxiety;
- low levels of energy, and poor physical recovery after illness or exercise;
- depression, and increased social isolation.

The symptoms and side effects of my brain injury were the same as the symptoms and side effects of high phe levels.

The effects of being off PKU treatment

I have never been completely off the PKU restricted diet therapy. But there have been months, even years, when I've not followed the regime closely. Even now, there are weeks when I will eat more protein than I am allowed. There are the odd days when I've missed supplements because life was just too hard, or too busy, or I simply couldn't face taking them.

In my first year of university, my supplement was delivered to my student hall on a monthly basis. One month, I noticed the colour on the packaging was a little different. But I was busy, so assumed it was another rebranding. It wasn't. The delivery company had sent the wrong supplement. I didn't spot this, and started taking the supplement for another inherited metabolic disorder. This supplement contained phe.

It was grading-week, and I was busy with exams, lectures, playing football, and generally being a normal student. It took me five days to notice the mistake. By then, my grade average had gone from an A- to a D. My lecturers couldn't explain the change, and nor could I. I was emotional, confused, and furious with everyone. I had fallen out with all my friends. A sobbing mess trying to work out what was wrong.

Dramatic deterioration, prolonged recovery

Once I noticed the error, the guilt, shame, and anxiety I experienced were devastating. I was alone, and crying down the phone to my mother at the other end of the country. The pharmaceutical company made an emergency delivery that day. I was back on the correct supplement and receiving emergency advice from my clinic within hours. But, while the change was dramatic, it took much longer for me to recover from the high blood phe levels.

This is something reflected in the findings of the team at Birmingham Children's Hospital when they studied the effects of the first restricted diet therapy. To prove their diet worked, they needed to conduct a double-blind test on Sheila Jones. This meant that, unbeknownst to the Jones family, they swapped the supplement to one with phe.

Sheila's condition deteriorated dramatically within a few days. However, once she was returned to proper treatment, it took much longer for equilibrium to return to her blood phe levels, and to her behaviour.

From my personal experience, I have found that however long I'm off the diet for, it takes roughly twice as long to recover. However, this isn't universal! People who returned to treatment after years report improvements almost immediately.

My finding is only a personal rule of thumb, and my PKU is severe. Just as everyone's PKU is different, so is their reaction to, and recovery from, high blood phe levels.

I do not recommend deliberate experimentation to find out your personal recovery time. However, on an occasion when you may have strayed from the diet, perhaps pay attention to how long it takes for you to feel normal again.

Returning to PKU treatment, it is never too late

It is never too late to return to PKU treatment.

People who have spent years away from PKU treatment have found changes and improvements within months, or even weeks, of returning. If you have been off diet for years, do not feel that you will need to be on diet for the same length of time before you see any benefits.

If you have PKU, and are considering returning to treatment, I encourage you to read how others have found the return to treatment. There are links to support for returning to treatment in the *Resources* section. It is never too late, and you are never too old, to return to PKU treatment and start seeing benefits in the way you feel and think.

Hope for returning to PKU treatment.

You might read the above and think, 'if my brain is already damaged, how would returning to PKU treatment help?' The answer lies in the brain; more specifically, in the processes of neurogenesis and neuroplasticity.

Neurogenesis and Neuroplasticity

Neurogenesis

Neurogenesis is the process by which the brain creates new neurons. It starts when the embryo is just developing, and is a crucial process in the growth and development of the brain. Formerly, it was believed that this process of creating neurons stopped once we became an adult. But evidence emerged in the second half of the 20th century which showed that neurons could develop in the brain in adulthood. We now know that neurogenesis is active through-out our lives. The brain is always making new neurons.

Neuroplasticity

Neuroplasticity is the concept that the brain can rewire itself. Or, as a neurologist puts it, 'the brain can change in response to training' (O'Connor, 2020). Neurologists used to think once the structure of the brain and its network of connections had finished developing in our youth, that was it. That that was the full quota of brain cells and development we would ever get. From then on, it was down hill. Science and neurology has now largely abandoned this theory in favour of neuroplasticity.

You may have already heard of this, following the famous study on London taxi drivers which was reported a decade ago (BBC News, 2011). The brains of trainees were put through MRI scanners before and after learning 'The Knowledge'. 'The Knowledge' is one of the most demanding series of examinations in the world, designed to ensure that taxi drivers instantly know the fastest route through 25,000 streets in central London.

The scientists found that the gruelling process of study and examination had a structural effect on the brains of the trainees, which was visible on MRI. This proved that the brain could change in adulthood as a reaction to the tasks it undertakes.

PKU and mental health

Mental health and wellbeing is a vast and evolving area of research. It is accompanied by numerous stigmas. The mental health considerations for those of us with PKU come not just from the effects of high phe, but also from societal and everyday pressures which result from the way it is treated. For these reasons, I have dedicated a complete section to *PKU and mental health*.

Hope for recovery

While I was recovering from my brain injury, I was advised that most of the recovery would happen in the first six months. This was a throwback to the now out dated belief that the brain doesn't develop or change after a certain point. Neurogenesis and neuroplasticity disprove that. I have improved immensely in the eight years since my injury, and continue to see changes now.

This is why we manage PKU. Our brain is not a fixed entity. It will still heal and change itself, if we can only look after it. No matter how long you have been off PKU treatment, there is still hope for improvement on return.

7. What causes the symptoms of PKU?

The reason that people with PKU experience distressing symptoms is due to the higher levels of phe in their blood. But, why do high levels of phe cause these problems? Three mechanisms may be:

1. Phe toxicity.
2. Competition at the blood/brain barrier.
3. Disruption of neurotransmitters.

Phe toxicity

One of my electives at university was toxicology. It was a fun course, and involved experiments on consenting students (as it was ethically difficult to poison unknowing participants). The first lesson was anything can be a toxin at high enough levels. It is possible, though extremely difficult, to overdose on water (Farrell & Bower, 2003).

The elevated levels of phe in the blood of someone with PKU will translate across the blood/brain barrier, and result in higher levels of phe in the brain. When it is present in these abnormally high amounts, phe becomes a neurotoxin. That means it can directly cause damage to the brain. Getting to the bottom of exactly why and how high levels of phe can cause this damage is still a mystery to science. However, it has long been inferred that phe does act as a toxin, given the correlation between high blood phe levels and cognitive disabilities.

Aspartame: a word of caution. Aspartame is synthesised from two amino acids, one of which is phe. This is why people with PKU are not allowed aspartame, which is commonly marketed as NutraSweet, Equal, or Canderel. Aspartame has attracted controversy. There are many theories, some credible but many not, as to the effects of aspartame on the human body. It is worth bearing this controversy in mind if you plan to do any reading on the subject.

Competition at the blood/brain barrier

Phe is one of a group of Large Neutral Amino Acids, or LNAAs. If levels of phe in the blood are unusually high, the blood/brain barrier is flooded with many more phe molecules than normal. This increases the competition for passage across the barrier. That competition limits the amount of other LNAAs, nutrients, and essential chemicals passing across the blood/brain barrier. Research into this continues, but it offers an alternative treatment mechanism. (See *Beyond the restricted diet therapy*.)

The good news is that the PKU supplements may also provide competition for phe at the blood/brain barrier. Research has indicated that this effect also works for the newer supplements synthesised from GMP (Ney, et al., 2009). There is more in the chapter *Supplements in the 21st century*.

High blood phe and neurotransmitters

High levels of phe crossing the blood/brain barrier may disrupt neurotransmitters, like serotonin and dopamine. Serotonin may have a good influence on mood, emotion, and sleep (NHS website 2, 2022). Dopamine is sometimes called the reward hormone, as it has an effect on the brain's reward and pleasure centres (Lienard, 2018). Dopamine also plays a role in muscle control and movement (NHS website 3).

A note about research

In 1981, around the time my parents were learning how to wean a child with PKU, research found a deficiency in both serotonin and dopamine in PKU (Curtius, 1981). It is perfectly reasonable for any parent to have missed this. However, I was gobsmacked to come across this effect only while researching this book.

Forty years of living with PKU, and I'm only now understanding how high blood phe might alter some key neurotransmitters in the brain. It is partly my fault as I nearly studied dietetics, but instead took a degree in winemaking. It was the fun choice, and my parents were relieved. They didn't want PKU to dominate my life.

As I pointed out at the start, I am not an expert in neurology and neurotransmitters. The entire point of science is to continually develop new theories, while revising and refining existing ones. The finer details of understanding the brain is a work in progress even for experts, so this is a basic overview of neurotransmitters & PKU.

Do remember that the body does a good job of regulating neurotransmitters. For those of us with PKU, it is about ensuring that we supply our body and brain with the resources they need, while adhering to the restrictions of our PKU treatment.

Serotonin

Serotonin appears to have a role in modulating our mood, cognition, reward, learning, and memory functions, alongside other physiological processes in the body. High levels of phe have been shown to disrupt the function of serotonin in the brain, which in turn can disrupt mood, memory, and motivation.

Some symptoms of serotonin deficiency do align with the symptoms of high blood phe levels in PKU. These symptoms are from different sources, so are not exact alphabetical matches. The symptoms in italics are those which align across the table.

Serotonin deficiency (Lamoreux, 2021)	**Symptoms of high blood phe** (PKU.com, 2021)
aggression & impulsive behaviour	anxiety
anxiety	*behavioural or social problems (akin to aggression & impulsive behaviour)*
depressed mood	brain fog & slowed information processing
insomnia	*depression*
irritability	Difficulty with decision-making, problem-solving, and planning
low self-esteem	inattention
poor appetite	*irritability*
poor memory	*problems with memory*

Improving serotonin levels on the restricted diet therapy

Serotonin levels are one of the reasons why supplements are crucial on the restricted diet therapy. Serotonin is derived in the body from the metabolism of tryptophan (Jenkins, et al., 2016). Tryptophan is another of the essential amino acids which humans need, and must source from their diet. Many of the foods which are high in tryptophan are high in protein, and are restricted.

For those on the restricted diet therapy, the best source of tryptophan is the supplement. If your amount of daily exchanges permits it, then soybean and egg are also fairly high in tryptophan. This is not an option for me as my exchange allowance is low, hence an emphasis on taking all of my daily supplement.

Dopamine

Dopamine has a complicated role in the body, most of which is still being researched. It is known as the 'reward hormone' due to its role in stimulating repetitive behaviour by giving a 'buzz' as a reward. While that is widely known, research shows that dopamine has a role in many other functions. These include digestion, memory and focus, mood and emotions, sleep, and stress response (Petrangelo, 2019).

In PKU, a lack of dopamine may be more important than a lack of serotonin. This is because the body makes dopamine when the PAH enzyme breaks down phe. The amount of PAH and its metabolism of phe is impaired when someone has PKU. Hence, it is feasible that people with PKU will make less dopamine. There have been several studies into this, but there is a need for further work.

As with serotonin, some symptoms of dopamine deficiency do align with the symptoms of high blood phe levels. These symptoms are from different sources, so are not exact alphabetical matches. Again, the symptoms in italics are those which align across the table (next page).

Why do we manage PKU?

Dopamine deficiency (Petrangelo, 2010)	**Symptoms of high blood phe** (PKU.com website, 2021)
difficulty concentrating	anxiety
movement difficulties *	behavioural or social problems (akin to aggression and impulsive behaviour)
poor coordination *	*brain fog and slowed processing of information (akin to reduced alertness, difficulty concentrating)*
reduced alertness	depression
reduced enthusiasm	Difficulty with decision-making, problem-solving, and planning
reduced motivation	*inattention (akin to reduced alertness)*
	irritability
	problems with memory

A tremor is commonly reported among people with PKU, particularly with high levels of phe. This has been backed up by research (Pérez-Dueñas et al., 2005; and Nardecchiaa et al., 2019). Therefore, there may be more symptoms of high blood phe levels linked to dopamine deficiency: poor coordination, and movement difficulties.

Improving dopamine levels on the restricted diet therapy

Your body requires both of the amino acids phe and tyrosine to synthesise dopamine. Again, this is where taking the PKU supplements is significant. Supplements provide your body with the tyrosine it misses out on in the diet. Though, one food which is both high in tyrosine and phe-free is watercress.

It has been widely understood, especially during the recent pandemic, that exercise has a positive effect on mood via dopamine and serotonin neurotransmitters. Recent research in animals has shown that both exercise and music can indeed have an effect on the regulation of dopamine (Petzinger, 2015 and McGilchrist 2011).

Finally! Here is a double win for those of us with PKU, as exercise can have an effect on blood phe levels. This is important as it is a non-diet mechanism which has widely reported beneficial effects on our overall health and wellbeing.

There is more on this effect in *Blood phe levels and testing*, and in *Healthy eating and exercise with PKU*. As is always the case in science, more research needs to be done. But, perhaps we should all enjoy more exercise and music, ideally at the same time.

Last, but not least, there is research which suggests that the synthesis and effectiveness of dopamine may be affected by Omega-3 levels (Healy-Stoffel and Levant, 2018).

Eczema, skin repair, and Omega-3

Eczema is a common symptom of PKU, with many on higher blood phe levels suffering from this painful skin condition. My family first heard of a link between PKU and Omega-3 when I was in primary school. I had eczema behind my ears and under my eyes, which was both painful and unsightly. It was one of the things which prompted a visit to a clinic.

We discovered the link between the impaired metabolism of phe and a lower level of tyrosine. Tyrosine is involved in the repair of skin and ligaments, and low levels of tyrosine can contribute to delays in wound healing (Brown and Phillips, 2010). I still have scars from those periods in childhood when I wasn't taking all of my supplement.

To my parents' relief, and my chagrin, the grey sediment which had been settling at the bottom of my supplement, and which I had been avoiding, was both the problem and the solution. By avoiding that icky sediment, I was missing some amino acids which were critical to metabolism. One of those amino acids was tyrosine.

We were also advised that I should start taking fish oil tablets. This was the early 90s, and it was suspected that the oils in fish may have a role in skin repair, cognitive processes, and protecting the heart.

While researching for this book, I found that the greater body of research conducted in the last 30 years has been unable to prove a statistically significant benefit in taking fish oil supplements to treat eczema (Wollenberg, et al., 2018). It is likely, then, that my eczema was the result of my habit of skipping part of my daily supplement to avoid the foul flavours.

Tyrosine is one of the heavier amino acids, and the bulk of it would have precipitated out into this remaining sediment. Once we ensured that I drank all of the supplement everyday, the eczema soon healed and the condition of my skin improved. Personally, I do still take fish oil tablets, but only at the dose as worked out by my PKU clinic.

Tyrosine is also required in the synthesis of melanin. This may be behind the interesting and dramatic changes in hair colour where enzyme booster therapies like sapropterin are used. (More about sapropterin in *Beyond the restricted diet therapy*.)

Sleep and PKU

Sleep disturbances may be a hidden symptom of high phe levels in PKU. The NSPKU dietician noted, 'sleep problems are not one of the commonly reported problems with PKU. But when you specifically ask about sleep disturbances, it would seem they are not uncommon in the PKU community.' (Ford, 2022).

There is a dearth of published research into this specific area. However, a study conducted in 2017 found PKU individuals suffer more from sleep disorders, reduced sleep quality, difficulty falling asleep, and sleepiness in the day than those without PKU (Bruinenberg, et al., 2017).

The study also showed that the sleep quality in mice with PKU was detrimentally impacted. The researchers were able to draw a direct link between sleep disturbances and PKU. There have been numerous studies into the roles which serotonin and dopamine play in sleep quality and regulation. Though the mechanism of these transmitters is still poorly understood, it is possible that the effect which PKU has on serotonin and dopamine may be the reason for poor sleep quality.

A summary

When we look at the symptoms of high blood phe, we see that many of them relate to our brain. The brain is a remarkable organ, yet we know comparatively little about it; we aren't even sure what it is made from (Tompa, 2019). Neurological research is ongoing, and science learns more every day. All of these effects of PKU emphasise the need to manage PKU in our daily lives. How do we do that?

Part three: How do we manage PKU?

8. Blood phe levels and testing

There are as many ways to manage a restricted diet therapy as there are variants of PKU. The key is to manage your PKU, and not let PKU manage you. That is possible, though it is difficult at times. Hopefully, some ideas in this section can help, or give you ideas on how & where to find support.

Given the emphasis on blood phe levels in this book, it will be no surprise that monitoring blood phe is important. There are five crucial elements to managing PKU, which are:

- Blood phe monitoring,
- PKU clinics,
- PKU supplements,
- specialised PKU foods, and
- finding PKU-friendly foods.

Why is blood phe testing critical?

The main focus in treating PKU is to prevent damage to the brain caused by high levels of phe. At present, the best way to do that is to reduce the levels of phe crossing the blood/brain barrier. Current treatments do this by focussing on maintaining low levels of phe in the blood, and this means that blood phe levels require frequent monitoring.

Guthrie tests and blood spots

I wrote a little about the Guthrie test in an earlier chapter, and many people with PKU now call this the blood spot test.

The original name comes from its inventor, Robert Guthrie. This is another example of an invested parent furthering the science and treatment of PKU.

Robert Guthrie's second son developed cognitive disabilities. Though the family spent years searching for answers, a diagnosis was never made (Koch, 1997). This experience imbued Dr Guthrie with a life-long interest in cognitive disability. At the time, PKU was diagnosed either by the unreliable nappy test, or required a substantial amount of blood to be drawn directly from the patient's veins.

A colleague brought this to Dr Guthrie's attention, and challenged him to do better. It only took him three days.

Three days to develop a reliable test which could help thousands avoid brain damage. This test was developed 25 years after Dr Følling first used bacteria to discover the levels of phe present in blood. Dr Guthrie also used bacteria in his simplified method, one which will be familiar to those with PKU, and to paediatric nurses around the world.

Blood from a pricked finger, or a newborn's heel, is dropped onto an absorbent card. This card is sent away to undergo the technique which Dr Guthrie invented, a bacterial inhibition assay.

While the blood collection method has remained the same, bacterial inhibition assay has since been replaced with new analytical techniques, such as tandem mass spectrometry, or high-performance liquid chromatography (Gregory et al., 2007 and Jeong et al., 2013).

This Guthrie card, or dried blood spot card, is still used by those with PKU, and their families, to test blood phe levels on a weekly, or monthly, basis.

Dried blood spot frequency

The recommendation for how frequently to test blood phe levels changes along with life stages, and in reaction to life events. The European guidelines for PKU make the following recommendations:

- Age 0–1 year: weekly
- Age 1–12 years: fortnightly
- Over 12 years of age: monthly
- Maternal PKU: weekly before conception, increasing to twice-weekly once pregnant.

Blood spots can be another battleground for families who are managing PKU. The tests may be difficult for young children, or those with a phobia for needles. There are tips and tricks available to help, especially the NSPKU's informative 'Blood test advice' article which appeared in their magazine a few years ago, and is now available on their website.

Getting a routine for the weekly or monthly blood spot can be helpful. Adults should bear in mind that, while it is tempting to pick the first of the month, the fact that it might be a weekday or weekend can make it difficult to remember to take the test. However, that random nature is a point in favour of the 'first of the month' system. If you always do a blood test on a Sunday morning, how do you know what the levels are after a busy workday?

Blood result delays

This testing system was a considerable improvement for PKU diagnosis and monitoring. However, it is now sixty years old. One of the main problems with the system is the delay in receiving the results. Because the blood cards must be sent for analysis, these delays can be so long as to render the test irrelevant when living with PKU.

Through a long system of trial and error, I have worked out that if I do a blood test a certain day, then I usually get a result the next day. This is useful as I can often still remember any little snacks or treats which may have snuck into my diet two days previously.

However, this has taken years of experimentation to work out. And it depends on a significant number of variables involved in getting the blood card from me to the lab. Postal system delays, inaccurate sorting at the hospital, a change to the laboratory routine... All it takes is one small change, and a delay renders the result less useful.

That listing of possible delays may seem fanciful, but a longer delay is normal with PKU blood results. I invested energy into working out the best time to do a blood spot because, in the past, I have had to wait a fortnight for a blood result. Can you remember everything you ate and drank two weeks ago?

That length of time for a result is not unusual. Some people have had to wait up to three weeks. These results might tick boxes for clinics, but are not useful for someone attempting to work out if they are managing their PKU well. It would be incredibly useful to have a blood phe testing system which could be used at home for fast, and relevant, blood phe results.

Blood phe monitoring at home

Diabetics have been able to monitor their blood glucose levels at home since the 1980s. Diabetes is exponentially more common than PKU, and thus there is a larger market for at-home blood glucose monitoring devices. Though we are forty years behind, there is at last progress on a blood phe monitor for use at home.

In 2020, the National PKU Alliance showcased three companies in a webinar on home monitoring devices. This webinar is now available on YouTube (NPKUA, YouTube, 2020), and gives a patient-level overview into the challenges involved. The possibilities look exciting, with multi-device functionality and an app to store and share results safely. However, what we really want is something cheap, accurate, fast, and easy to use at home.

There are several challenges which need to be sorted out before any device can come into our homes. First, to measure the amount of phe in the blood, you need to find those phe molecules and distinguish them from all the other components in blood. The phe molecules are small in comparison with other molecules, so they must be marked by a reagent. This reagent highlights the phe in the blood, and helps the test to be both faster and more accurate.

The amino acid tyrosine is relevant to PKU because it is similar to phe. In this case, that similarity can cause problems, as tyrosine in the blood can be wrongly recognised as phe. This means testing methods may count tyrosine as phe, and thus give an elevated reading. This must be correctly managed in any home monitoring device.

It feels like we have been waiting years to test our phe at home; we have! However, there is progress. Several companies are now attempting to licence home monitoring devices in both the USA and the EU. These plans were delayed by the pandemic, but clinical trials are restarting.

In the UK, we are still awaiting treatments which have been in use elsewhere for years. Access to home monitoring on the NHS may yet be another battle for PKU campaigners in the UK. Note that the UK is no longer in the EU; meaning success on the continent does not guarantee treatments nor devices in the UK.

While researching for this book, I came across a paper which suggested that dried blood spots tend to underestimate blood phe levels. The researchers took dried blood spots and blood from the veins of PKU patients at the same time. They then compared the phe level results. The blood taken from the veins gave a higher phe level than the blood spot tests (Stroup, et al., 2016).

One paper does not mean we need a complete change. But it is possible that dried blood spots may not be the standard test in future. Most of the home monitoring devices in development involve dropping blood from a pricked finger directly into the machine. They no longer use dried blood spot cards. Hopefully, the removal of that step will result in more accurate blood phe results.

9. What else affects blood phe levels?

Restricting the amount of phe we eat is often the most effective mechanism we have to manage our blood phe levels. Unfortunately, the phe content of food is not the only thing which might influence blood phe.

High blood phe levels

Phe intake is the most likely cause of higher blood phe levels. But, if your diet has the correct amount of phe, and the products you eat or drink have not changed to use aspartame or high-protein ingredients, where else can you look?

Not enough food or supplement

The next likely cause of high blood phe levels is that the body is not getting enough nutrition. The PKU restricted diet therapy involves a balance between the nutrients provided in foods, and those provided in the PKU supplement. Not eating or drinking enough of either could mean that the body is not getting the nutrition needed to grow.

A metabolism which is not getting enough energy and nutrients from food and PKU supplement, will attempt to find them elsewhere. This can lead to a process called catabolism; where the body starts to break down its tissues to release protein and nutrients into the blood stream. It was a drastic form of catabolism which caused the sudden weight loss and high blood phe problems during the creation of the initial PKU treatment (Green, 2020).

If the body is breaking its protein down, this will release amino acids from body tissue back into the blood stream. Some of these amino acids will be phe. This will cause high blood phe levels, even if the amount of natural phe eaten in the diet hasn't changed. If this is the case, it is important to make sure you are taking all the PKU supplement which your body needs, and have enough phe-free food in your diet.

I agree, it can be awfully difficult to take all the prescribed amount of supplements. If it is not proving possible to take the full amount of your current supplement, perhaps it is time for a new flavour, or an entirely different type of supplement. The technology behind PKU supplements has changed markedly in the last decade. There may be one more suited to you, and I discuss supplements later in this section.

If your prescribed amount of supplement has not been checked recently, or if you are taking all of your supplement but still have high blood phe, it is worth having the calculations run again. I used to think this was a simple calculation of body weight and phe tolerance, but it isn't. That is why the best person to check your supplement amount is a trained metabolic dietician or health professional.

You can access these specialists though a clinic, and this is one of the most important reasons to go to a PKU clinic. Attending a PKU clinic can be an unwelcome experience. I have written more about clinics and steps which might help in *Making PKU clinics work for you*.

Decrease in rate of growth

A slowing of growth as children and teenagers age may cause an increase in blood phe levels. This is one of the reasons that blood spots are recommended more frequently for children and teenagers, than for adults.

As a mother's growth requirements also decrease following the demands of pregnancy and breastfeeding, this change can be reflected in blood phe levels. Again, this is why regular blood phe testing in maternal PKU is essential.

Illness

Someone fighting an infection or a disease may need more energy than normal. Additionally, some forms of illness also lead to a reduced appetite. This may cause the body to go, temporarily, into the same catabolic process discussed above. Thus, when someone with PKU is fighting an illness, their blood phe levels may rise.

Exercise

Cardio exercises may be described as catabolic, where your body is breaking down tissue (hopefully fat!). It is possible that this same process of catabolism may cause blood phe levels to increase following intensive periods of cardio, repeated consistently for weeks. Do note that the intensity of exercise needed to have this effect is significantly more than suggested in daily exercise guidelines.

I could only find one research trial on blood phe levels after exercise, which showed no statistical difference in PKU patients (Mazzola, 2015). The European PKU guidelines stated that regular exercise in people with PKU must be ensured. There was no mention of the effect on blood phe.

The authors noted that the guidelines did not make a recommendation for high-level sports, as this has not been studied (van Wegberg, MacDonald, and Ahring; et al., 2017). Those were the only two mentions of exercise in the full guidelines.

For other recommendations, we must rely on our own anecdotal evidence. This is not ideal, but I do provide some in the chapter *Healthy eating and exercise with PKU*. Hopefully, more research on the effects of exercise in PKU will be forthcoming.

Menstrual cycle

The effects of the menstrual cycle on PKU are understudied, but there is a small amount of evidence for an effect on blood phe. Please see *Women and PKU* for more.

Low blood phe levels

We need to ensure that the level of phe in the blood is just right, not too high nor too low. There are several reasons why blood phe levels may low.

Growth spurts

Blood phe levels may be decreased by growth spurts. A fast-growing body will be using phe quickly to build new bone, muscle, and tissues. This is one reason why blood spots are recommended more frequently for children and teens, than for adults.

Pregnancy

The need to supply all the resources required by a growing baby means that the mother's blood phe levels and phe allowances need to be closely monitored during pregnancy. The increased demand means that blood phe levels may decrease rapidly. This means that the amount of dietary phe and supplement needed during pregnancy can increase dramatically. For more on pregnancy, see the chapter *Women and PKU*.

Exercise

As noted above, extreme levels of cardio exercise may cause elevated blood phe levels over a long period of time, e.g., weeks or months. Likewise, it is possible that the opposite type of exercise, anabolic or weightlifting, may reduce blood phe levels because the body is taking phe out of the blood to build new muscle.

Additionally, someone who mixes both types of exercise frequently for months on end may see their blood phe levels decrease through the same mechanism. The prolonged exercise is causing phe to be used to build stronger bones and muscles.

It would take quite a bit of exercise over a long time for this to be the main cause of low blood phe. As an example, I have played football for the women's reserve team of a Premier League club. There was a game every weekend and two weekly training sessions. Moreover, we were expected to train on our own to maintain our fitness. My blood phe levels from the time were at the low end of the recommended range, but were not exceptionally low. I did ask about it in clinic, but there was no sign that that level of exercise caused a problem with drastically low blood phe levels.

Lessons from 40 years of blood spot levels

On a personal note, I spent the formative years of my education following the stricter blood phe ranges required in Australia & NZ. At my last clinic session before emigrating to the UK, the clinicians advised that the UK diet is more lax than in NZ. They warned me to take care of my levels and keep them in the NZ range.

I'd like to say that I followed their advice. But I felt relieved, let off the leash a little! I made myself a personal limit, one in between the two differing ranges. My preferred upper limit for blood phe was 480 µmol/L. That was based purely on the desire for a less restrictive diet when I came to the UK. After researching for this book, I will endeavour to keep my blood levels in the 120-360 µmol/L range.

As anyone dealing with the PKU restricted diet therapy will know, that is not a simple goal. I spent a rainy weekend going through years of blood phe level notices and put them into a spreadsheet. Now I have a handy, and objective, record of my adherence to the restricted diet therapy going back to the age of 5. Out of 300 blood spots, my blood levels have been within the 120-360 range 65 times. That is 1 in 5 bloods.

That may seem disheartening, but looking back over the records showed me two crucial facts.

1. It is possible to get blood phe levels within that range, and
2. I usually achieved those levels when I had been exercising frequently.

This is something which has been commented on by other people with PKU. I have written more about this in *Healthy eating and exercise with PKU*.

10. Making PKU clinics work for you.

The environment in a PKU clinic can be make-or-break when it comes to sticking with PKU treatment. For the patient and their family, it might feel like you are being told off every six months, or having the headmaster check your homework. The attitudes on both the clinician and patient side are key to making a PKU clinic work at its best.

PKU is one of hundreds of inherited metabolic disorders (IMDs), which means that even those health care professionals running an IMD clinic may not often work with PKU patients. Those clinicians have guidelines to meet, tests to arrange, results to assess, and boxes to tick. That is alongside their primary focus on the patient.

A clinician may also approach PKU, or any IMD, from an objective viewpoint. One where the answers are black and white: you must do this to avoid brain damage. This is true, PKU and its untreated effects are serious. It is also true that the clinicians and dieticians need to have a human understanding of the daily struggle with PKU.

A friend has been studying nutrition to become a dietician. When we spoke, I joked about how she would discover how much I strayed from the diet. In response, she exclaimed that she had just been reading about how many people do not follow the recommended treatment.

My response was emphatic:

"Yes because it is so hard! You've seen all the effort that I need to put in, and all the effort you must go to when hosting me for a single night. Yet, I often have patches where I struggle with the restricted diet therapy. Remember those daily efforts when you are in clinics with your patients".

When attending a clinic, it may feel like there are some who see only the PKU, not the person. As the patient, you are the reason everyone is there. The person with PKU is the most important person in the room. Make the clinic work for you. To help with this, it may be a good idea to take someone supportive with you to the appointments.

Putting the patient first

There are many dieticians and health professionals who do attempt to understand the struggles of living with PKU. I have been with my PKU clinic since emigrating to the UK over a decade ago, and have a good relationship with them. I know from speaking to others that I'm fortunate in that. If you are struggling with your clinic, the section *What if the clinic isn't working?* may help.

In the last few years, my clinic and others have reached out for patient perspectives of PKU to share among their team. This pivot to discovering what life is like on the other side of the consulting desk is most welcome.

A dietician's focus on PKU may be a purely objective one focused on brain damage, amino acids and nutrition inputs. They may see patients once every few months, or less, so how do they see the daily perspective? How do you explain living with PKU to someone who approaches it from a medical or academic perspective? And how often has someone with PKU wanted to say: "If my diet is so simple, then you try it!"

Several people have stepped up to the challenge and done just that. In 2018, the NSPKU set out a 'Diet for a Day' challenge and convinced several politicians to try it. One of the UK Members of Parliament, Liz Twist, did complete this challenge while campaigning for PKU in parliament. The experience brought home to her the challenges which people with PKU face every day.

Before that, in 2015, I was glued to the blogs when registered dieticians Louise and Sarah undertook their '7 day 7 Exchange Dietitian Challenge'(Dietician's Life, 2015). Qualified dieticians with years of experience in the UK health system having to deal with the intricacies of a daily PKU diet? Yes, please!

There was a bit of pleasure from someone else's misfortune, but I am grateful for their explanation of the difficulties encountered, and for the tips they uncovered.

Making effective use of your clinic

People with PKU have fully trained, professional, and experienced dieticians on call. We should use them.

I have consulted my PKU clinic when I wanted to bulk up for a sport, and then when I wanted to lose a bit of weight. They have assisted me in my recovery from brain injury, and from sporting injuries. A six monthly consultation with trained dieticians is not something most people have. It is worth making the most of it.

It can be beneficial to take some time, even just five minutes, to think about the appointment before you are sitting in the waiting room. The key question is:

What would help you to manage your PKU?

- If you are struggling to take supplements, can the clinic team arrange for samples of a different type to be sent to you?
- If you are finding it difficult to stick to your phe exchanges, can they suggest some protein-free foods which might help to fill you up?

- You may have questions about PKU itself, such as how the blood phe levels might be affecting you in work, or at home.

Every so often, it can be helpful to have a list of what you are currently eating and drinking through the day. You may have already been asked to complete a food diary and send it to your clinic before the appointment. This can help them to answer your questions, and the preparation may allow them to support you more effectively.

Or, you may be embarking on something new, such as a new school, or preparing for a holiday. How can the clinic help you with those? You won't know unless you ask.

You may want to keep your PKU, and the clinic, away from other parts of your life. But PKU is a part of your life and the health professionals in clinic may be able to help you in the wider world too. This could be as simple as providing a letter to certify that any supplement in your luggage is a medical supply, which can help at customs.

Things to think about before your PKU clinic:

- Can a family member or friend go with you? They may feel more able to ask for an explanation, and can offer you reminders and support during the clinic.
- Prepare a list of the foods & supplements you are taking, and when you are taking them. Do you have enough to ensure a small surplus, or do you run out each month? If so, can the allowance for this item be increased?
- Do you have a list of questions or concerns ready? Order them so the most important is first. Ask if there are new products or treatments available.

- Do you need more lancets or cards for blood phe monitoring? Do you need any new shakers for supplement? You may not leave the appointment with these, but your clinic could still help you to access them.

What if the clinic isn't working?

The PKU clinic is meant to be a support for someone who is managing PKU. Somewhere to have questions answered or to receive advice. It should be a partnership focussed on the best possible outcome for the person with PKU. If your clinic hasn't felt like that, then there are options.

Support

If you feel unable to raise your concerns directly during the clinic, then the hospital, or health provider, will have a liaison service. In the UK, there is a Patient Advice or Liaison Service (PALS) for each hospital in all four nations of the UK. PALS offer a point of contact, and confidential advice and support, including on a formal complaint procedure.

Patient charity and advocacy organisations are another source of advice and support. The NSPKU in the UK have already helped people with their PKU clinics, and helped improve the professional-patient relationship. If you are having problems, I urge you to get in contact.

Change

If these pathways do not change how you feel you are being treated at your PKU clinic, there is the option, at least in the UK, to change your PKU clinic. This is possible, and I know of several people for whom this has worked. I have managed to do the opposite. When I moved out of the catchment area, I requested to stay with my current clinic, as I felt supported there. I was granted permission, and my appointments have continued as normal. The main point is that, whether clinic is working for you or not, then there are options out there and people who can help.

It may also be worth taking time to think about how you approach the clinic. Do you walk in ready for a confrontation? Or are you just going to say whatever you need to say to just get out of there without feeling attacked or rebuked?

Health professionals don't want you to feel like this either, though they may not realise that they are causing it. Take time to think about why you feel this way, is it frustration with the diet, or with feeling ashamed when discussing difficulties, or that your efforts are not being recognised?

Dealing with PKU is hard, and exacts a heavy mental toll on the person with PKU and on those looking after them. This is why the PKU clinic should work with you, part of your tool box. If you pick up that tool in dread, then no-one is getting the best from it.

Perhaps before your next clinic, take time to think about how you feel and why. And you may realise that it is time to seek advice on how to change that feeling. This is diving into the mental health toll of PKU, which I discuss further in the section on *PKU and mental health*.

Returning to a clinic or changing to a new one

In the UK, the best way to return to PKU clinic is via a referral from your GP. Elsewhere, it is best to check the *Resources* section for information relevant to your area.

If you want to find out more before taking that step, most national charities have a confidential helpline which you can call. They might help you with questions and to find out more about changes in the treatment of PKU where you are.

Food diaries

These can be another point of conflict with a PKU clinic, and a source of frustration or shame for the PKU patient. A food diary is a list of everything you eat and drink, including supplements. Most food diaries carry across several days, usually a week, to capture different activities and meals. They can feel like a chore, but they are useful.

A food diary will give both you and the dietician a decent overview of your whole diet. The food diary isn't merely a check on if you are sticking to treatment. It is about ensuring you aren't missing any important nutrients, and that the diet is balanced. The time that you eat both your natural phe exchanges and your supplement is significant, especially with exercise.

Even if your diet hasn't changed much at all, it may be worth doing a food diary to be sure that everything you need in your diet is there; and in case something which shouldn't be there has crept in. It is easy to stray and pick up a hidden exchange or two over time. I know, I have been caught out several times when I thought that nothing had changed.

The key to keeping a food diary is to make it work for you. That may mean that you make a note on your phone each time you eat or take a supplement. Or you take a photo of the packets with a note of how much of each food you ate. Or you may already plan your PKU restricted diet for the day or the week on a board in the kitchen. Take a photo of that each day.

Food diaries must record what you are actually eating. I'm afraid that there is no point in not being honest on food diaries, you are only hurting yourself.

Yes, I've done a food diary at Christmas. Yes, I ate too much protein. But I told the dieticians, and they helped me to work out which treats were better for me than others, and which treats I should really be staying away from. The next time we had a party, I was able to eat more food, and have more treats, with less guilt. It worked!

We have experienced dieticians on call. Use them.

11. Supplements: a key battleground

Supplements are one of the three keys to the PKU restricted diet therapy. They are also one of the main battlegrounds. The reason for the struggle is taste.

Taste, or flavour, is what dieticians mean when they refer to palatability. How something tastes is key to whether someone will be able to eat or drink it. That is as true for a 4-month-old as for a 40-year-old. It is difficult to force yourself to take something regularly if it is not an attractive flavour.

Taste can also refer to an aesthetic, rather than palatability. This is also key for supplements which need to be portable, as well as potable, and discrete enough to fit into the lifestyle of someone with PKU.

Palatability of Supplement

This is one of the main reasons people struggle to take their supplement. A survey held by the NSPKU in 2018 found that 11% of children with PKU were either not able to take their full supplement dosage in a day, or were not taking any at all (Ford, 2018). That figure increases with age, and 58% of adults with PKU were not taking the supplement, or were unable to take the full prescribed dosage.

Nearly half of PKU patients cannot follow the full treatment. And those who can, rarely enjoy it. The survey also asked why people with PKU found it difficult to follow the PKU restricted diet therapy. The palatability of the supplement was in the top three reasons for both children and adults.

The reason for the challenging taste of the amino acid formula is the flavour of the individual amino acids themselves. Many of these are bitter and unpleasant. The first supplements were a combination of essential amino acids, vitamins, and minerals. Strong flavours are needed to mask this combination of unpleasant flavours.

Spare a thought for those making the supplement. To be useful in any way, our medicine must contain some pretty foul tasting components. On a PKU study day in London in 2018, the Nutricia product development team demonstrated this by asking delegates to mix their own 'amino acid supplements'. The results were enough to make everyone present a little more grateful for the efforts put in by flavour developers.

The good news is that there are now supplements which use a different source material to create the PKU supplement. These are widely reported to have an improved flavour with less bitterness. If you are one of the many who struggle with the amino acid-based formula, find out more in *Supplement in the 21st century*.

Early PKU supplement

The first experimental supplement for PKU was synthesised by the team at Birmingham Children's Hospital in the early 1950s. (See *Pioneers of the First PKU Diet* for more details.) As the entire venture was theoretical at that point, palatability was not a consideration during its development. The formula was a mix of amino acids and essential vitamins which had been filtered out of a milk protein.

Anne Green's book *Sheila* tells this lost tale with aplomb, and describes the difficulty in administering the formula to the first restricted diet patient, Sheila. Getting supplement into children has been a battle ever since they were invented.

The formula became commercial soon after its development. Several companies began to make a low-phe or phe-free formula for the treatment of PKU. This was the beginning of a new era in the treatment of both PKU, and other 'orphan' disorders.

Orphan disorders are those rare disorders which require treatment, but which are so uncommon individually that the market for any treatment is not large enough to either gain support or attract the resources needed to develop it. Despite these challenges, new drugs for orphan disorders are occasionally developed. Any drugs for these orphan disorders are known as an orphan drug. PKU is one of the few orphan disorders with any form of effective treatment.

Following the breakthrough at Birmingham Children's Hospital, there was suddenly a therapy for a condition which had previously been considered untreatable. The focus was to get a therapeutic supplement into the hands of newly diagnosed babes as swiftly as possible to prevent brain damage. It is hard to argue with that, and to insist that taste should have been their key concern.

Development of supplement in the 20th century

By the 1960s, supplements were established as a medical therapy. The next development in PKU restricted diet therapy was the creation of the phe allowance and exchanges. This helped to increase the variety of the diet, and provided more support to patients and their families who needed to follow the treatment outside the hospital walls. Given the wide range of foods which now had to be analysed for their phe content, supplement development was no longer a priority.

Older adults with PKU will remember the formulas from those days. These came as a powder in large tins. The dosage was measured out and mixed with water to be taken as a drink or a paste. It is likely that memories of the flavour hang around longer than the brand names of Minafen, Lofenalac, and Albumaid XP.

This last of these was developed in the 1960s, and was the first supplement for PKU from a company called Scientific Hospital Supplies, or SHS. This name may be familiar, as the company became well known for the products it produced in the late 20th century for metabolic disorders.

They were the first PKU supplier I knew of in the 1980s, indeed the only supplier I knew of until returning to the UK in the 21st century. Through a series of mergers, SHS became Nutricia, and the company is still the source for the bulk of my supplement and other prescription foods.

Maxamaid XP and Maxamum XP

Like many people of a certain age who have PKU, the first supplement I can remember was Maxamaid XP. This was the next-generation supplement from SHS, following on from Albumaid XP.

Maxamaid XP was the first phe-free drink with a deliberately added flavour (Wikipedia, 2022). However, Maxamaid XP was not the first supplement I was on. Babies and young children tend to switch supplement more frequently than adults as their needs change, and as they are weaned.

Partly because of the lack of choice available in New Zealand at the time, I remained on Maxamaid XP from toddler to teen. The change from Maxamaid XP to the new Maxamum XP came when I was 13. And it proved to be quite a difficult switch. Having become accustomed to one supplement, the alteration in flavour was a tough one to stomach. Not that there were many options. I had a choice of orange flavour or unflavoured.

Having tried, and failed, to make a palatable PKU supplement myself, I must state that I am hugely grateful for the work which nutritionists and product developers did with a challenging formula. That said, those who smelt these supplements often asked me to describe the flavour. Over the years, I honed my responses as follows:

- Maxamaid XP: Like a fermented orange curry
- Maxamum XP: Like used football socks left in a hot car

My family employed a variety of tricks to encourage me to drink my supplement, a battle which any families managing PKU will be familiar with. One of the best, which I still remember, was a special cup used solely for my supplement. This cup was purchased while I was a toddler, and it worked so well that it was still in use during my primary school years.

It was a reusable form of the smoothie cup which you find frequently today. But in the domed, see-through lid was a little merry-go-round with four ponies. The merry-go-round mechanism linked to the straw. The faster you drank liquid through the straw, the faster the ponies in the lid would turn. Even now, my aunties remember encouraging me to 'make the ponies go faster!'

That cup was a work of genius. Turning taking medication into a game, was a winner. I treasured that cup, and it lasted for years, travelling the world with my family. But eventually, it broke, and I haven't seen one since.

Measuring older supplement doses

Maxamum XP, and the other older supplements, were supplied in bulk tins with a 50ml scoop. The scoop was used to measure out the powder needed for the supplement each time. I remember needing 3 scoops of powder per drink.

Taking a drink with each meal meant I was drinking 450 ml of the powder each day. Or attempting to drink. Because we would make this drink up before school, my lunchtime supplement would sit in my bag in an NZ summer for several hours before I drank it.

I soon found that the heavier amino acids settled out of the drink, leaving a greyish sediment at the bottom of the container. If I didn't shake the bottle well, that sludge would stay, and the remainder would taste better.

My attempt at skipping the more unpleasant flavours wouldn't last long. When I returned home, mum would add water to the bottle and mix it. Then I would sit on an actual naughty step and wasn't allowed to move until it was all finished.

This heart-wrenching battle, of a parent making their child do something horrid for the good of their health, is familiar to every parent. But parents of PKU have to face that battle all day, every day.

As an adult with PKU looking back on those days after several decades, I can tell you that it was worth it. I appreciate that may be cold comfort to those struggling now. The good news is that supplements have changed dramatically since then.

12. Supplements in the 21st century

If you abandoned your PKU supplements over a decade ago, or have been struggling with the same one for years, then it might be time to look again. While taste was rarely thought of during the development of the first formula, supplements have undergone a dramatic transformation.

Taste, both in terms of palatability and aesthetics, is now a key consideration when companies develop their PKU supplement. There have been marked advances in the way the dosage is worked out, as well as in the supplement format, presentation, and source material (or what they are derived from).

Working out supplement dose

Whoever thought up this new system of arranging and packaging the supplement dosage deserves a medal. Today, the standard practise is that PKU supplement comes in different packets with numbers on them. E.g. PKU Air 10, Sphere 15, Lophlex 20.

The words are the different brand names for each product. The numbers refer to the amount of amino acid equivalent provided in each packet. Amino acid equivalent means the equivalent amount of natural protein supplied by that pack of supplement.

So, in the examples given above, PKU Air would supply the same amino acids as someone would get if they ate 10g of natural protein. The Sphere provides 15g, and the Lophlex gives 20g.

Before researching this book, I assumed that the amount of supplement someone required was a simple calculation of their body weight and how much protein they were allowed. I had made this calculation myself a few times. However, I was wrong!

The amount of supplement which someone needs is derived from several factors:

- severity of PKU, i.e., how much phe the person can tolerate;
- stage of development, e.g., those with growth spurts may require more;
- the person's lean muscle mass, not simply their weight.

Given the complications involved, it is always best to ask a clinic or a PKU health professional to work out your supplement amount.

I discussed some problems with clinics in *Making PKU clinics work for you*. But even if the only advice you are prepared to take from a clinic or specialist is your supplement and your phe tolerance, then please ensure you get these calculations done professionally.

Supplement format

You can still have a supplement powder which you mix with water, or another liquid, to drink. These tend to come in single-serve sachets now, which are easier to carry and use than a bulk tin. Or you can cut out the tap and have your supplement delivered as a ready-to-drink liquid. Again, these tend to come in a single-serve pouch or carton.

In my trials of new PKU supplements over the last decade, I have tried a pudding type supplement which you eat with a spoon. Some companies offer the supplement in tablet form.

I did use these for a while, but found that you had to take a lot of them.

Some tablets were available as a flexible set, where you could decide if you wanted to have that particular dose of supplement as a tablet, a drink, or eat a bar similar to a cereal bar. I loved those bars, as they felt like a snack and a supplement in one. Sadly, they weren't popular, so were discontinued. There are other companies who now produce the supplement in a bar format, and I'm hoping to get a taster pack soon.

Another form of supplement is the granular supplement. Essentially, the supplement comes as tasteless granules which you sprinkle over a meal and eat without even noticing it. This was interesting, but leads to the problem of 'you have to eat everything on your plate!' This can be difficult for adults as well as children. Who among us hasn't over-filled their plate at a buffet? At the time of writing, this type of supplement was available with a recipe book which suggests methods of working the supplement into food and drink.

A newer format of supplement is something called 'micro tabs'. These are tiny tablets, but not as micro as granules. Their size reminded me of the sweet (candy) 'Nerds', though micro tabs are uniform in their appearance. They were also tasteless, though it was hard to tell as they were to be swallowed immediately with no chewing.

Micro tabs are taken by the capful, and it was handy to carry round just tablets and a drink bottle for the day. They were an interesting experiment, but not for me. And that is fine, I'm aware that micro tabs have worked wonders for other people with PKU. Bottom line is that there is a wide range of PKU supplements available now.

I would encourage people on the restricted diet therapy to contact their dietician about tester packs for different supplements. Experiment and try them. Supplement needs to be something that works for you and what you are doing. I have tried many formats, but keep returning to the powder sachets, as these work for me. But it is always worth trying something new, as it might be a better fit as your life changes.

Supplement presentation and aesthetics

The format and source of the supplement are about palatability. Presentation is where the aesthetic comes in. Supplement needs to be in a format which you feel comfortable with, but also presented in a way which doesn't discourage you from taking it.

I used that odd double negative of 'doesn't discourage' for a reason. It can be hard to be positive about PKU. I recall being in a focus group for a company which was asking about attitudes towards a nascent PKU product. The group facilitators were puzzled by the lack of 'very positive' responses on the attitude grid. I spoke up with "but that's how things are. I don't leap out of bed every day thinking, \Yes, I have PKU!' It is just something you deal with in the least negative way possible".

The presentation of the supplement covers both how it is packaged, and how it is branded. Both of these do have an effect on how willing someone with PKU is to carry the supplement away from the home, and to drink it when around other people.

Growing up in NZ meant you had to get sun-smart quickly. There was a debate about the best type of sunscreen, whether lotions in a squeeze bottle were better than roll on, or if we should be using sprays; whether sunscreen in makeup was as good. I'll always remember what a sensible person pointed out: it doesn't matter what format something is in if you don't use it.

Basically, use the format which suits your lifestyle, which is easy for you to carry around and apply. The same applies to supplement.

It doesn't matter whether your supplement comes in a snazzy sachet or a tin, a juice box carton, a tablet bottle, or a pouch. If the format means you can't carry it with you, or that the supplement is difficult to take, then try another format.

Make your supplement work for you

I know some people who take their morning supplement warm in a reusable coffee cup. It works for them, and other people assume it is their morning cuppa. Some people prefer to drink their supplement straight from the fridge. Another PKU person I know mixes their powdered supplement with two or three times the suggested amount of water. This dilution means they can sip it from a water bottle, and everyone carries one of those these days.

The trend for people to mix and take supplements or electrolytes after an exercise session also helps people with PKU to blend in. Nobody in my gym batted an eyelid when I stopped to mix up a powdered drink after a workout.

This trend has also led to improvements in the mixers available to those who take a powdered supplement. Bottles with a separate compartment to keep the supplement powder dry until it is needed are now common place. Though, it is easier and cheaper to use the ones which are usually provided free with the supplement by the manufacturers.

I have used these bottles for other things too. The addition of a device to aid the mixing of the supplement also helps to remix a home-made smoothie. This makes for an easy, protein-free or low-phe snack while out and about.

As mentioned above, some different supplement formats are designed to work together. For example, Nutricia make several supplements under the name 'PKU Lophlex' which are designed to work together to give you options for taking your supplement. You might prefer to mix a powder drink in the morning, take a ready-to-drink pouch with you during the day, and eat a pudding like supplement in the evening. There are options which let you chose a mix of tablets and powdered drink.

It is OK to try something, then stick with what you know

I have tried all these formats, but still stick with the powdered drinks. The single-serve sachets make the powered drink format far more attractive than the bulk tins ever did. Being able to simply put a sachet and a mixer in the bag, then take it later without the bother of scooping or weighing makes a big difference. I am concerned over the waste, but so are the companies who develop these, and they are working on recyclable packaging which maintains the viability of the formulation.

The sachets of powder also work well when I travel. The new formulation means I can carry all my supplement for a three-week holiday in my carry on luggage, which is reassuring. The tablets were also easy to travel with, but I found them less kind to the stomach after a beer. There is more on travelling in *Travel & emigrating with PKU*, and a little on the in's and outs of alcohol in *Celebrations with PKU*.

Online forums for PKU are a good way to find reviews of available supplements, but I do urge you to try new items out yourself. What doesn't work for someone else, may work for you, and vice versa. Clinics are the best place to get your supplement dosage worked out, and to arrange trial packs and new prescriptions. Another good source for advice is the websites of the companies which make the PKU supplements and prescribed products. (There are links in *Resources* at the end of the book.)

Glycomacropeptide, or GMP

Until the 21st century, all PKU supplements were the same, a mix of amino acids and added flavouring. By 2008, a new way of making the supplement had been discovered.

GMP is a protein which occurs naturally in cheese whey. "Great," you say, "but we can't have cheese." (Or "Grate, but we camembert it." I know, I'm sorry.) However, when GMP is extracted from cheese whey, it is a dietary protein which is naturally low-phe (Ney, et al., 2009).

GMP has a minimal amount of phe, it contains 5mg per gram of protein. Or there is 0.5g phe in 100g of GMP. In the UK, this amount is considered to be phe-free for people on the PKU diet.

In the first decade of the 21st century, researchers extracted GMP from cheese whey and used that as the basis for a new amino acid supplement. Initial tests on mice, which were genetically altered to have PKU, showed that the new GMP formulation had no immediate adverse effects. However, it is important to bear in mind that GMP is not completely phe-free. More about that below in *Cautions needed with GMP*.

Tests on humans with PKU followed, and almost immediately the increase in palatability was noted during the research trials. This led to an increased adherence to diet, and hence to an improved clinical outcome. Basically, the GMP supplement tasted better, which meant it was easier for people with PKU to take all the required dosage, which led in turn to lower blood phe levels.

This was the first major advancement for the palatability of PKU supplements, since the addition of flavouring to create Maxamaid XP over 20 years previously. Vitaflo were the first to bring a GMP-based PKU supplement, 'Sphere', to the UK market in the 2010s.

In the short time since, the number of GMP-based supplements available has multiplied. GMP was first available as a powdered mix to blend with water. There are now GMP-based ready-to-drink supplements, and bar formats too.

Benefits of GMP

Taste

The increased palatability of GMP-derived products is a big win. It has proven key in helping some people with PKU adhere to the restricted diet therapy. In addition to the increased palatability, GMP may offer other improvements.

Hunger and heartburn

I've been fairly lucky with my supplements in the past, but one of my current treatments does give me gastrointestinal problems fairly frequently. This can be as much of an issue much as flavour and convenience. When a medicine makes you feel worse, one is much less inclined to keep taking it, no matter how it tastes.

Trials to date suggest that GMP can improve these gastrointestinal issues, and help you to feel full (Ney, et al., 1026). Anecdotal evidence from both my testing and the PKU community agrees with this claim.

Lower cost

One of the studies into GMP reported that the lower cost of making this type of supplement means that the treatment might become a more viable option in developing countries (Zaki, O.K.). I did not expect to be counting my blessings while researching for this book. But I am lucky to have been born, and resided, in countries which have the expertise and resources to diagnose and treat PKU.

Cautions needed with GMP

While these possible benefits make GMP appear spectacular, there are several cautionary notes to bear in mind.

Phe content

As noted above, not all the phe is removed from GMP. In 2020, a handbook produced to support dieticians, nutritionists, and physicians cautioned that when GMP is used for all the supplement, it can increase the blood phe levels in children (MacDonald et al., 2020).

This reflects the fact that, while the amount of phe in each supplement sachet is small, it becomes significant if many supplements are taken over the day.

As an example, Sphere is one of the earliest and more common GMP supplements. One packet of Sphere15 contains 28mg of phe, or just over half a UK exchange. The Sphere20 contains 36mg of phe, or about 3/4 of a UK exchange.

This fact led me to believe that if I changed all my supplement to Sphere, I would be having about 140mg of phe from supplement. That's nearly 2.5 exchanges, or half of my daily allowance! (Note: 1 UK exchange is 50 mg of phe, a US exchange is 15 mg).

That concerned me because I assumed that it would be a straight trade-off. That the amount of phe in my supplement would be deducted from my daily phe allowance. This meant it was 18 months before I decided to try a GMP supplement. My PKU clinic said that it was unlikely that the phe in a GMP supplement would directly translate to higher blood phe levels. But the only way to find out, as with so much of the PKU restricted diet therapy, was to try it. Basically, to conduct a phe tolerance challenge on myself, using the GMP supplement.

On the suggestion of the PKU clinic, I monitored my diet closely and did blood spots before starting, and again after two weeks of trying the GMP supplement. I was expecting high blood phe levels. I had already resigned myself to thinking that, while GMP was the tastiest supplement I'd come across, it was sadly not for me. However, a scientist would say, "never speculate ahead of results."

When the blood phe results after the two week GMP trial came in, I was rather chuffed. The level was well within the European guidelines, and also within my own personal range, denoting where I feel best. While you need to be aware of the extra phe in GMP supplements, especially if you have classical PKU, this does not mean you cannot take GMP.

Reported benefits not all in humans

Some benefits remain unproven in humans: while there are examples in the PKU community of GMP supplements improving satiety (filling you up) and reducing heartburn, these have yet to be proven in large trials.

It seems appropriate to end this section on GMP with the cry of scientists across the ages: more data is required!

Supplements in a nutshell

The two key things about supplements are:

1. Take them

Please take them! Even if you have gone over your phe amount that day. In fact, especially if you have gone over your phe amount. They may help your body to absorb and limit the damage by reducing the amount of phe crossing the blood/brain barrier. Supplements also provide most of the extra nutrients you need to keep feeling well. You don't have to love supplements, not all medicine can be helped with a spoon full of sugar, but some supplements genuinely are nice.

2. Have them with meals

They are supplements, meaning they are there to help nourish you. Supplements do their job best if you have them when you are digesting other food. It just means your body has everything it needs to hand. Also, they help to fill you up.

Mix and Match

It may have taken you a while to find a supplement which you can stomach regularly, and you prefer not to switch. That is fine, but equally you don't need to switch to simply try something new. Most large supplement companies offer trial packs, so you can try their different supplements at home.

You might prefer several flavours of the same supplement. Or could end up having the same flavour across different formats, as a powder, as drink ready to go, or a pudding pot. The point is to try them. PKU conferences are a good place to do this, or you can order them to try at home.

I noted that I stick with a powder supplement because this works for me. But I don't have the same brand. I actually take two different supplements from two different companies every day. This give me a little variety. One of the supplements is an amino-acid formulation, while the other is a GMP. This provides extra variety, even if they are both powder formats.

Remembering to take a supplement

I take four supplements a day, with breakfast, lunch, dinner, and the last as an afternoon snack. But there are days when it doesn't work like clockwork. I might miss one, so end up having two supplements at once. No, that isn't the advised way to take them, nor is it pleasant. However, I do feel better than if I miss one out entirely.

Carry it with you

To that end, I carry my supplement when I go out. Because I take a powder supplement, this usually means sticking a sachet in a mixer and buying or carrying a bottle of water. If you use the ready-to-drink types, or one of the bar formats, this is even easier. I also have a spare sachet which lives in my bag in case of emergencies. This gets swapped out every few months, when I remember to do it.

Prepare the daily dose

Every morning I get out the four supplements and put them on the kitchen counter, or on the bedside table if I'm travelling. That way, I will not have to remember if I've had them all. If there is still one on the bench or the bedside table, I'll take it before bed. That feels like an old-school method now, as I came up with it before the smartphone existed.

Reminders

Setting reminders on our phones or watches is another good way of remembering to take the supplement. Ideally, supplements should be taken around meals, but this means we might feel uncomfortably full. If this is true for you, then setting an alarm for an hour before or an hour after eating is a good reminder.

There are apps to help track supplement and phe allowance every day. I didn't think I needed one until I tried it, and discovered that I was exceeding my phe allowance. It was only a little, but a little every day adds up. This is also where a food diary might help to spot the little extras which creep into our diet. (I have written more about food diaries in Making PKU clinics work for you.)

Supplement delivery

Both of my different supplements are delivered to my door which makes it easier to manage stocks. Several companies offer this option, check out the specialist supply companies near you, there are some links in Resources at the end of the book.

13. Focus on food

The PKU restricted diet therapy may seem all about food, it certainly feels that way when we are hungry! It might be considered unlucky that it is chapter thirteen which finally discusses food, but there is help out there.

Specialised PKU foods

Once the specialised medical food companies had released their first PKU supplement in the 50s & 60s, they turned their attention to substitute foods. The first foods were designed for the basics in the diet; protein-free milk, and a bread substitute. The bread used to arrive in tins.

Now, several companies are making substitute foods for those on the PKU restricted diet therapy. These companies range from giant multinationals, to small family companies who were inspired when their family members received a PKU diagnosis. While there are still substitutes for the everyday basic items like bread, milk, and pasta; the variety of foods available has expanded to include biscuits, chocolate, crackers, and convenient snack pots.

In the UK, and some other countries, PKU substitute foods are available with a prescription from a central health service. In other nations, e.g., the US & Australia, these foods must be paid for, either on insurance or out of your own personal pocket.

Furthermore, the variety and availability of products for PKU can vary across both countries and time. For these reasons, I recommend sourcing current availability from your clinic, or check the companies near you. There are a few links in the *Resources* section.

Home delivery services for PKU supplement and foods

For years, I was collecting my supplement and foods from the local pharmacy. This was fine in NZ, when I had a car. Following my move to London, however, I was car-free, and needed to carry boxes of liquid and food on public transport. Every so often, I needed to make several trips to collect it all. Clearly something had to change.

At one of my clinic visits, I discovered that some companies who make the items also have a home delivery service in the UK. I will admit that signing up took a bit of time and, of all things, a fax machine. But that was a decade ago, and for the last ten years all of my PKU supplement and foods have been delivered to my doorstop every month.

This has meant that managing the PKU diet is far less hassle. Depending on the service you use, the company may also liaise with your GP over prescriptions. I fill out a form, or receive a phone call, and the company arranges the prescriptions. Then, I open the door once a month to receive all the food. If you have a local delivery service, and some places have several, then I would urge you to try it.

PKU-friendly foods and food shopping

It is easy to become a creature of habit with the restricted diet therapy. The preparation and planning involved in managing PKU is exhausting. When you find a method, and a few meals, which work for you, it is common to stick to those routines.

Any changes can cause heightened anxiety at the prospect of not being able to eat, and requires expending more energy to make new plans. This same anxiety and stress over a change, or even the prospect of a change, may be present when we are working with new recipes or changing supplements. The anxiety may also appear over temporary changes, like a holiday.

Eating the same food daily, becoming a creature of habit, can help with the planning and preparation needed when managing PKU. And there is nothing wrong with good habits and strong routines. But equally, it doesn't mean that a change is automatically a bad thing. As an example, the explosion in plant-based foods for vegans, vegetarians, and those looking to reduce their impact on the planet, has been a boon for those on with PKU.

Finding foods

Wherever and however you shop, there will always be a lot of label reading. Every product intended for the person following the PKU restricted diet therapy needs to be checked to ensure:

1. It does not contain any item on the "red| forbidden list.
2. If it contains any ingredient(s) from the list of restricted foods*, that the intended portion size will be within the phe allowance.

The list of restricted food, and how much of that food counts towards the daily phe amount, is slightly different for each country. I discuss this in Restricted diet therapy today, *but do check with your clinic or specialist.*

Whether you are shopping online or in the store, every product will need to be checked. It is one of the reasons I prefer to shop online. But I am privileged in both living somewhere that the service is available, and being able to meet the minimum spend for delivery.

Suitable products

Once you have spent time checking each label, it is understandable that the same product ends up in your basket each shop. Buying the same brands may avoid the need to check ingredients and protein content. This is a key reason why those catering for PKU become creatures of habit. It is also why two of the most dreaded words for someone with PKU is "new recipe".

Manufacturers may justify changes to a product's recipe as a bid to reduce sugar, or to improve flavour. This may cause problems for those with PKU if the change results in the use of, or an increase in, those ingredients which contain protein. Or with a switch to aspartame to reduce sugar levels (*see below*.)

There are sources of information which can help people to shop for PKU. In the UK, the NSPKU provide downloadable lists of the many phe-free, or low-phe, foods available in the major supermarkets. The *Resources* section has links for these, and for the US, Australia, NZ, Canada, Ireland, and other European countries.

Another source of information on new foods suitable for PKU is the PKU community. In the last few years, the online community for PKU has introduced me to new yoghurts, 'sausages', ready-to-eat dessert pots, and easy-melting 'cheese'. I have written more in the chapters *Community and Support* and *Tell someone that you have PKU* about cultivating an online PKU support community, and this is one of the key reasons to do so.

Aspartame in foods

The focus on sugar content over the last few years has had some negative effects on foods available for PKU. Both the change in public attitudes to sugar, and the imposition of sugar taxes has led to an increase in the use of artificial sweeteners.

While most artificial sweeteners do not cause problems for those with PKU, aspartame must be avoided. Phe is one of the main ingredients of aspartame, making it toxic to someone with PKU.

Aspartame has been one of the most popular artificial sweeteners for decades. NutraSweet was aspartame, and the branded trademark popularised its global use and familiarity.

The risk which aspartame poses to someone with PKU is recognised. In the EU, any product containing aspartame must highlight the fact under the ingredients list. Usually, under the list of ingredients, a label will carry the phrase 'contains a source of phenylalanine.'

In other countries, aspartame may simply be listed in the ingredients. It may even be listed without a name, but as the **additive E951**. When shopping for PKU food, drinks, and medicines, the labels and ingredients lists must be scrutinised for these signs.

Costs of PKU-friendly foods

In the UK, the cost of both the supplements and prescribed foods for the PKU restricted diet therapy are covered by the NHS. It is worth remembering the same is not true for other countries.

If I lived in the US, the cost to my insurance company of the yearly supplement alone would approach USD15,000. This is approximately GBP11,000 at the time of publication. (Cost in 2021 from US prescription price comparison site Script Save Well RX, and the exchange rate from XE.com.)

While we contemplate the elevated cost of supermarket shopping for someone with PKU, it is worth remembering the true economic cost of PKU restricted diet therapy is higher. That said, the personal expense of PKU-friendly foods from the supermarkets and grocery stores is considerable. Low protein versions of everything from staples to luxuries always cost more.

From a monetary perspective, the cost of PKU-friendly foods is a massive burden. The NSPKU have reported the cost to the NHS of the prescribed foods to be up to £16,000 per patient every year. Families and individuals with PKU must spend considerably more than the average food bill for PKU-friendly food. The following examples show that PKU-friendly foods can cost two to four times more. (All costs are from a mid-level UK supermarket in June 2021).

Example: A coconut-based plain yoghurt (160g is 1phe) costs 40p/100g. That is four times more than the cost of normal plain yoghurt, which is too high in protein for someone with classic PKU on restricted diet therapy.

A person on the restricted diet therapy needs to pay three or four times more than others simply to have yoghurt. I would argue that the costs of the PKU diet and its effects must be included in any cost-effectiveness study, because it is a prescribed treatment for an inherited metabolic disease. Food is used as a treatment for PKU, therefore the cost of specialised foods should be considered as a healthcare cost.

Financial assistance

Around the world, people with PKU may be eligible for assistance with the costs of the restricted diet therapy. Given the requirements and processes for these payments changes across nations, any information printed in this book will soon be out of date. The *Resources* section has some links which were accurate at the time of publishing, or approach your local PKU support group.

14. Living with PKU, a personal story

While I did attend school in the UK, I did not have to deal with school meals for long. When I was 5 years old, my father realised his life-long dream of emigrating to New Zealand. In the pre-internet 1980s, New Zealand really was an unknown, far-a-way place. However, houses were sold and bought, new jobs found, boxes packed, and goodbyes said. And then we were off. Just Mum, Dad, brother, sister, and me against the Orcs of Middle Earth.

Daunting as this was, there was also the problem of finding support for a PKU diet at the other side of the world. All the prescription foods and supplement had to be shipped in from overseas. With the strikes of 70s Britain still in their minds, my parents reconfigured the cupboard space in our kitchen to hold a 3-month supply of all my supplement and food.

This was less of a difficulty than you might think because the variety of PKU foods available was decidedly limited. Along with my supplement of Maxamaid XP, we received flour mix and pasta spirals. That was it.

Essentially, I lived on fruit & veg, the PKU pasta spirals and whatever new ideas my mother could craft the PKU flour into. More recently, new bread makers and recipes have made PKU loaves a joy!

Other varieties of pasta shapes, the PKU cereals, cookies, snacks, and crackers were not available in NZ until I was in my late teens. Fortunately, we lived in a part of New Zealand known as the fruit bowl. Avocados, melons, and kiwifruit were plentiful, alongside the more typical offerings of apples and citrus fruit.

As noted before, while I have tried to remain 'on diet', I haven't always been a patient in a PKU clinic. Our rural NZ settlement was a five-hour drive from the nearest PKU dietician.

When I was 6, my mother and I left home at 3am to make the journey. Thanks to traffic it turned into a 12-hour round trip which was not a great experience. Because of the distance, and just life in general, I was next seen by a dietician 10 years later, at the age of 16.

For the decade between 6 & 16, my 4 exchanges allowance of phe remained the same. In my early teens, a series of letters (this was pre-email) suggested an increase in my supplement. I went from three icky supplement drinks a day, to six. There was one at breakfast, three in my school bag for lunchtime and both morning and afternoon breaks, then two more in the evening.

I spent a lot of time on the naughty step after school trying to finish the grey precipitated remnants in several drink bottles. This was not easy on my parents, but their relentless struggle to keep my PKU on track was worth it.

There were social challenges too. I went to a tiny school, which had only 25 students. That wasn't the number in my class, that was the total number of students in the entire school. There was nowhere to hide my restricted diet therapy, blending in at lunch times simply wasn't an option. So, I had to go the other way and tell everyone I was actually an X-Men reserve. Only not all mutants have super-powers.

I'm aware that I was bullied over my PKU, though I remember little of it. I realise that it will be of cold comfort to anyone going through it now. But it is more important for your future to stick to the diet in school than to worry about what people think.

I know that isn't helpful at all. Just like when others tell you that those jibes which hurt so much, or the people who are making your life a misery, will not matter in another few years. That is all well and good, but they certainly matter at the time.

But, your brain matters too. As does your body. In a few years, when the bullies or the not-quite-friends have gone to a different school or disappeared from your life, you will still have your brain and your body. They are with you for your entire life, and they are worth taking care of. Now, many years on, my mother remembers the bullying while I do not.

I graduated into high school, where I was in the first 11 football team, the string quartet, the drama club, and the top quartile of scholarly achievement. If that sounds like showing off, it is for a good reason. Those of us with PKU may be told that we will not be able to achieve the same as others, or that we will be slower, or more frail.

This does not need to be true! You can be a high achiever, and have PKU.

My parents were told not to expect much intellectually from me. And that I would likely struggle with exercise and co-ordination. This was forty years ago, and only 30 years after the discovery of a PKU treatment. We now know a lot more about the outcome of treated PKU.

How did my parents deal with the devastating news that they needed to have low expectations for their child? They simply didn't tell me. I was unaware that I wasn't supposed to do well at school, so I went ahead and did well anyway. I didn't know that my hand-eye co-ordination was supposed to be too poor to play a musical instrument or participate in sport, so I did both anyway. It is remarkable what you can achieve when you aren't aware of the limited expectations which others have for you.

Along with leaving the bullies of primary school behind, another big change while attending high school was that the world was opening up. The primary schools were small village affairs, and my parents worked in the same town. High school was in a city, 35 miles (56km) away from home.

The move to a large school was a bit of a wake-up call for my parents. In only five more years, if all went to plan, I'd be leaving home for work or university. There would be many new responsibilities, alongside significant change. It would be quite a burden to manage, and there would be unknown challenges.

The one thing my parents could prepare me for was the management of my PKU. It was this realisation, along with the precursors of teenage behaviour, which showed my parents I needed something every teenager wants more of: control. And, if I learned how to manage my diet in my teens, it meant that when the time came for me to leave home, there would one less thing for all of us to worry about.

I already knew a fair bit about my diet, how much phe I was allowed every day, how much supplement I had to take, and how to weigh it out. Now the challenge was to make sure I understood why the diet was important, as this would give me reason to follow it.

My parents encouraged me to explain PKU when we met new people, they would only step in when I got lost in the terminology. This helped me to understand the need for a restricted diet therapy, and reinforced how essential the treatment was.

I began tracking my supplements and planning my exchanges through the day. This meant that if I wanted to eat my lunch during morning tea time, I could do that. But I also learned that it would make a lunchtime without a phe exchange more difficult. And the temptation of extra chips from the canteen soon faded when my parents helped me to see the connection between them and the headache which interfered with the fun of football practice. It was a delicate line between letting me learn from my mistakes, and keeping control for themselves.

It paid off, though. After two years of managing PKU restricted diet therapy on my own, my parents and I both felt confident enough to send me on an outstanding 3-week school trip to Japan. No parents watching over my shoulder, only a few teachers who were in charge of 15 other students at the same time. Would I cope?

There were mistakes, but not massive ones. I stayed away from everything on the red list. There were some days when I ate more rice than my phe allowance permitted as my diet was mostly rice, seaweed, pickles, and beans.

But I stuck to the supplements and indulged in light-hearted bargaining with my friends. "How about four of your pickle nigiri for two pieces of my steak?" It is these small things that helped both me, and my friends, accept my diet as normal. Something to be lived with rather than battled against.

I should perhaps note that my school did not usually send students to Japan for school trips. This opportunity was a combination of connections through our Japanese teachers which kept costs down and a year of fundraising by our entire Japanese class. The added incentive was that it was 50 years since the first atom bomb exploded over Hiroshima. We were to pay our respects at the peace park as part of our trip.

I came home with memories which have lasted a lifetime, and a new confidence in my ability to manage PKU. Since then, I have always been on the PKU restricted diet therapy where-ever I have travelled. It is possible!

A few years later, I left home for university to study the fabulously titled Bachelor of Viticulture and Oenology, or grape-growing and wine making. Yes, I had found a way for the university to subsidise my alcohol consumption. I discovered I quite liked this, so went on to a career in the wine trade.

It wasn't all plain sailing, but a return to a PKU clinic helped. Since we had managed to navigate the twist and challenges of PKU with no clinic input for a decade, you might think: "why come back to clinic?"

I was moving out of home to a different area of the country with a new health system. The PKU clinic smoothed bureaucratic waters and offered valuable support with sourcing supplement and foods. Clinics can be helpful places. It may not feel that way, you might still feel very much like you are being told off sometimes, but hopefully that is something else that you can change.

My journey with PKU is not over, and new PKU treatments are in development as I write this book. However, nobody knows what the future holds, and this is especially true for those with PKU. It is now 70 years since the development of the restricted diet therapy, but "diet-for-life" has only been in practice in the UK since 1993.

There are many adults with PKU who no longer follow the restricted diet therapy, or who have returned to treatment after they followed the earlier clinical advice to leave. There are also few older adults who have remained on restricted diet therapy for life.

This means there is a dearth of information on the effects of life-long restricted diet therapy as people grow older. This is an area where I have been pushing for more research and information, and I hope to have the answers soon!

Part four: PKU and mental health

15. Research on PKU and mental health

The initial research into PKU centred on finding a treatment, rather than on the palatability of any therapy. Similarly, the study of the PKU restricted diet therapy has focussed on the physical and neurological effects, rather than on the emotional or mental health of PKU patients.

This reflected the urgent need to treat the physical symptoms, including the clear evidence of cognitive disability, in those with untreated PKU. It also reflected the attitude of society at the time.

A good start

In the last few years, new research and treatments for mental health conditions have helped to bring a focus on mental health issues in wider society. There is still a long way to go in both treating mental health conditions, and in removing the surrounding stigma. The change is welcome, and has led to a more open discussion of mental health in those with PKU.

Mental health isn't as obvious as eczema, but living with PKU does affect someone's emotional state. I confess to a reluctance in writing this section on PKU and mental health. It involved exploring some areas of the PKU restricted diet therapy which are uncomfortable and difficult for someone with PKU to face, even if they are currently on treatment.

Furthermore, a person's reaction to the strain of a PKU diagnosis and the required treatment will vary, as will any possible remedies.

PKU and mental health

This reluctance to discuss an aspect of PKU was unusual for me. Since childhood, I have always been open about PKU and the difficulties it causes. My first speech on PKU was in the debate forum at high school, and I have discussed PKU at events, magazines, and, now, a book.

I was once invited to speak to young adolescents with PKU about the transition from paediatric care, to PKU care as an adult. As part of my preparation for the presentation, I asked PKU families and adults on social media what they would have most liked to learn about PKU when they were of a similar age.

One of the responses was:

"Tell them what we all want to know, in life as well as in PKU. How you deal with that question: 'What Went Wrong?' How do you banish shame, guilt, anxiety about mistakes; whether they were accidental, or if you knew but didn't care at the time?"

Wow! If I had the answer to what we all want to know in life, I'd market it for millions. The truth is that almost nobody's life is as good as they make it out to be. We all have our struggles. But, just because today didn't go well, it doesn't mean that tomorrow will go badly too.

Personally, I found dealing with my diet anxiety much easier after learning a bit of mindfulness meditation. I've written about that in *Anxiety and PKU*. But, what worked for me may not necessarily work for someone else.

This section explores some mental health issues encountered when living with PKU, and possible coping methods. The first step is to understand the problems.

Current research into mental health and PKU

The causes of depression and anxiety are many and complex. Those experienced due to PKU, and the restricted diet therapy, are no exception. There is now a growing recognition that prolonged exposure to elevated blood phe levels may still occur even when following the restricted diet therapy. Further, these higher levels may cause a higher rate of 'mood disturbances' than there would be in the general population (Clacy, Sharman, & McGill, 2014).

These 'mood disturbances' include depression, anxiety, and stress. It is true that this was a tiny study, the trial only involved eight people. However, PKU is so rare that we are never going to have the luxury or reassurance of data from high participation trials.

Another paper (Bilder et al., 2017) had similar examples of neuropsychiatric co-morbidities, which included anxiety and depression, as well as eating disorders and cognitive dysfunctions. That paper then investigated the prevalence of these mental health problems in patients with PKU. Finally, the researchers compared those rates to the prevalence in both the general population, and in people managing diabetes.

The review found that while people with PKU have a higher prevalence of these identified conditions in comparison with the general population, the instance is in line with that found in the diabetic group. Both groups are dealing with the social exclusion and extra planning which happens when a medical condition is treated through the severe restriction of foods. It stands to reason that both groups would suffer similar mental health complications.

Results from a large survey on PKU

Another source of data on the effects of PKU on mental health comes from one of the largest surveys of people living with PKU (Ford et al., 2018). The paper reports that there were 631 participants, giving us an unprecedented insight into the lives of those with PKU. And it provides a meaningful quantity of data for statistical analysis.

Along with depression and anxiety, this survey showed that many people with PKU struggle with low mood and indigestion problems. Parents reported that a third of children with PKU had difficulties in education. Also, one third of adults with PKU reported difficulties in gaining qualifications, or with career progression.

Eating disorders

The same survey showed that some people with PKU have an abnormal relationship with food. Half of all adults in the survey reported trouble with their weight, or suffered from abnormal eating patterns, or eating disorders.

This is not unexpected. Food is being used as a medical treatment, so it is not surprising that those on the restricted diet therapy have an unusual relationship with food. But, of serious concern, is the fact that only 4% had been able to receive treatment for their eating disorders.

Social Isolation

Food is a sociable activity in many cultures. However, those on restricted diet therapy are excluded from some of the activities centred around food. Meat is not allowed, which makes it difficult to fully participate in the Sunday roast or the Christmas turkey.

While there have been advances in the availability of vegetarian and vegan options, and in society's acceptance of these dishes; this does not mean catering for PKU is easy. Those who must restrict eggs or nuts cannot simply have the quiche or nut-roast option. Again, half of those responding to the PKU survey reported experiencing social isolation because of the PKU restricted diet therapy.

A need for support

These are all indications that those with PKU would benefit from specialist support. Similar support is already available to others with long-term medical conditions, or who are undergoing treatment for cancer or major trauma. A recent article in the NSPKU News & Views (Turland, 2021) focussed on how the complex management of PKU might be supported by a clinic team which had a greater understanding of the psychology involved.

The author of the article is a trained clinical psychologist who has studied anxiety and depression in diabetes. She is now part of the PKU community following the diagnosis of her child; and expresses her disappointment that a psychologist was not already a member of the PKU clinical team and called for that to change.

The benefits which the support of a clinical psychologist provides for diabetes, and other long-term conditions, has already been recognised. Sadly, this is another case of those with PKU and rare diseases needing to fight for the same recognition as other conditions.

While the active PKU community campaigns for such support, and other treatments what can we do now?

- We can attempt to understand the emotional burdens of living with PKU, and how these might affect us.

- The PKU community can support others with PKU. Non-judgemental support from someone who understands what living with PKU is like can be incredibly helpful.
- We can, if we feel ready, set out to improve the awareness of PKU in society and health care, which might help us now, and in the future.

The emotional burden of PKU

The emotional burden of living with PKU may manifest in various ways. This list is not exhaustive, nor exclusive. Someone who is attempting to manage the PKU restricted diet therapy may struggle with several of these problems at once. Or they may be living with other PKU-related issues which are not covered in the following chapters:

- *Anxiety and PKU*
- *Social Isolation with PKU*
- *Abnormal food behaviours from PKU*
- *PKU, depression, and fatigue.*

Remember that the physical effects of high phe appears to include disruption of neurotransmitters. This may be a cause of anxiety or depression. If you need help with the emotional burden of PKU, please speak to your clinic, a professional, or someone you trust.

16. Anxiety and PKU

Anxiety is one of the main mood alterations found in studies on people with PKU. Sadly, PKU may predispose us to be anxious due to the effect which high phe levels have in the brain. I've written more about this in *What causes the symptoms of PKU?*.

PKU means managing your food all day, every day. It means working out how to get in your supplements while finding the 'Goldilocks' protein zone — not too much phe, not too little. When you add in the need to find specialised PKU products and suitable groceries, it's not surprising that food can become a considerable preoccupation.

As if things weren't bad enough, we live in a society where food is cast as a weapon or a medicine, a panacea or the cause of all illness. You need only glance at social media, and news headlines to see how much judgement and scrutiny is devoted to ordinary diets. Food can be classed as healthy, unhealthy, processed, natural, junk...

Now consider that the current treatment for PKU is all about controlling what you eat. I have lived with PKU for over 40 years and am an active member of the PKU community. I go to conferences, clinic days, cooking demonstrations, and I do not believe that I have ever met anyone with PKU who doesn't suffer from food anxiety. Over time, I have realised that I also have food anxiety.

People with PKU tend to be anxious about our food. Food may be a threat to us. But equally, we require food to survive, and it is an integral part of societies and cultures. We are automatically excluded from many rituals and celebrations. Christmas dinner is fun, but with a twinge of sadness and isolation, as we can't try everything on the table. Try living with that and not having mental and social complications.

The unknown losses, and the known worries

At the age of 11 I missed out on 100% in a science test because I was unable to identify a substance. It was milk. Because I couldn't drink milk, I wasn't familiar with the smell and was unable to identify it.

This was a single mistake in a single test, which I happen to know about because I asked the teacher afterwards. This mistake clearly occurred because of my PKU. But in the last 30 years, how many other tests were failed, opportunities lost, mistakes made, or social occasions missed because I carry this burden through no fault of my own?

And living with the uncertainty, anxiety, and frustration of those losses, well, it is slightly similar to what everyone else has had to live with during the Covid-19 pandemic. Only PKU is for a lifetime. We need to learn to manage our anxiety.

Personal experience with anxiety

I'm lucky in that my personal situation has been stable for a few years. This has combined with efforts in my childhood to mean that my PKU has also been stable. Unlike many of my generation, my parents made the difficult decision to keep me on the restricted diet therapy when UK policy recommended that treatment could stop.

While I wasn't taken off the diet, I have most certainly wavered and had months (years) where I did not stick rigidly to the treatment. Now, I like to think that I have a healthy attitude to the odd treat and low-phe day to make up for it.

Note that the method of a day of excess followed by a day or two of extra restriction is not recommended by clinicians. It is simply how I cope with the restricted diet therapy in the real world, the world with food-based celebrations like birthdays and Christmas.

A handy spreadsheet shows that my blood phe levels have been within the 2017 European guideline range for the last 5 years, with few exceptions which I can still name. The excesses were caused by birthdays & holidays with all their treats, and the need to navigate meals on planes or in airports.

And yet, I still have this diet anxiety. Anything can trigger it, but diet anxiety usually shows up when I go outside my usual routine. New events need a plan, and I won't be relaxed about them until I've found a few safe meals and mentally packed my supplement. I guess that I'm not alone in being a PKU adult who still worries about where their next meal is coming from.

My diet anxiety used to occur more often than it does now, and it affected me deeply. I would be in a flood of tears and rage about how damned unfair it was that no-one else needs to check out local menus before clicking 'buy-now' on a holiday deal.

In the midst of one of these episodes, I realised they were the same feelings I'd had a year before, triggered by similar holiday-shopping. At that point, it seemed useless to keep raging. Ultimately, the wailing didn't change anything and just wore me out.

Mindfulness

I later discovered that this recognition is the first step in a mindfulness technique. Mindfulness feels like it is everywhere now, and I used to think it was a load of twaddle for people with the luxury of time. But after a serious health problem, which wasn't PKU related, I was looking for anything which might give relief for a minute or two. That's when I found the RAIN technique.

R — Recognise: Realise and name your emotions e.g., anxiety, anger, or sadness.

A — Allow: Allow yourself to feel, it is normal to occasionally feel strong emotions.

I — Investigate: Why do you feel this way? What has triggered these feelings?

N — Non-identifying: Realise that feelings are part of you, but not all of you. Occasionally, you will feel strong emotions. But they are temporary.

This technique doesn't work universally — there is no single cure for everyone! However, it can provide a little space from whirling emotions, and help you to get back to a calmer place.

It helped me to accept that PKU is a part of me, which means that the anxiety will pop up from time to time. The key is to recognise it, and encourage it to fade quickly. I am more than my PKU. It is just something to be considered and allowed for in my life.

Pause the anxiety treadmill

You'll note that I've used the word 'pause' there. That is because it is impossible to avoid anxiety in everyday life, there will always be worries and concerns. But we might find ourselves stuck on an anxiety treadmill. Maybe sticking to the restricted food list has been really difficult for a while. Or we've been doing our best and just missed the aspartame in a drink.

Either way, it can be frustrating when you wake up with a headache, or brain fog. You might find yourself grinding through the familiar emotions of anxiety and blame. Thoughts can spiral around:

"What happened? Why am I feeling like this again? What did I do wrong, what happened?..."

There will be times when your investigations are successful; perhaps the cause was a simple change in ingredients. But on most occasions it will not be that easy to solve. If you were busy, or have been struggling for a while, then answering these questions might not be easy, or useful.

In these situations, continuing to search for an elusive answer can lead to more anxiety, feeding the cycle and just making you feel more guilt. If there ever was a time to be kind to yourself, this is it. Take a breath and realise that mistakes do not mean you are a failure. Be kind to yourself.

It was in the midst of one of these episodes that I picked up a mindfulness app and found the RAIN technique. Listening to a 5-minute recording didn't solve the problem at the time. But it did give me space to allow the anxiety to drop, and to think about the problem calmly. Over time, I was able to stop anxious moments without the recording, just by taking a breath and reminding myself of the technique.

So, that's it then, easy? Of course not. It is about pausing the anxiety cycle, not stopping it. This isn't a miracle cure to anxiety, just about giving you a bit more space to step back and breathe before starting again.

Occasionally, this technique isn't enough, and this is where it might be worth searching for some professional help. I have turned to both professional and volunteer counselling services in the past. It is nothing to be ashamed of. My only wish was that I hadn't waited so long. It is easy for anxiety to become overwhelming. And it can turn into, or appear alongside, social isolation.

17. Social Isolation with PKU

In many cultures, social occasions often involve food. Being able to eat the same food with another person has been a method of establishing a connection for millennia. To break bread with someone has social and religious connotations. Throughout human history, food has helped to encourage a sense of belonging, a shared commonality between people.

What happens when you can't share the bread?

This is one of the most common shared experiences, yet it is not possible, or is awkward and difficult, for someone on the restricted diet therapy. And, through no fault of their own, someone with PKU is automatically disadvantaged when a social occasion involves food, as most do.

This feeling of being placed on the outside of a group can be remedied, but it takes effort. The multiplication of this required effort across numerous social occasions can be draining, and enhance the feeling of isolation.

Friends and family can help ease this feeling through simple gestures, such as catering for the person with PKU, just as you would cater for a guest with diabetes or another medical condition. This doesn't have to be difficult, and I have made suggestions on how to do so in both *Planning with PKU*, and *Celebrations with PKU*.

Be assured that any small effort will make a big difference to the person living with PKU. Catering for someone with PKU is easier these days, thanks to the increase in the commercial availability of foods which can be adapted to the restricted diet therapy. It is not all sugar and roses, though.

Fad Diets & PKU

The prevalence of lifestyle diets in society exploded in the 2010s. It has become common for my friends or colleagues to discuss the merits of the keto vs paleo diets, or to inform a waiter that they are now gluten-free.

This increase in popularity and variety of diets in the wider public is both a burden and a boon for someone on a medical diet therapy. With more people asking about ingredients in shops or restaurants, we are somewhat less of an oddity.

However, the prevalence of new diets undertaken for lifestyle reasons can reduce the public's tolerance for those which are followed as a medical requirement. If many people are demanding information or food with extracted ingredients, there is less patience or sympathy around for those on a prescribed therapy.

I cannot be the only person with PKU to have explained the diet therapy restrictions to a new acquaintance only to inspire a rant: "vegan this and gluten that, it is all nonsense". Then, after a long pause, "not that your thing is nonsense, of course". Hmm.

The privilege of choice

It may be that an exhaustion of choice is behind this reaction. As supermarket shelves and menus fill up with more brands or ingredients, it becomes harder to find favourites or to make a simple choice. This choice overload (Reutskaga et al., 2018) is a studied phenomenon. It is linked to decision exhaustion, otherwise known as simply giving up on deciding at all (Cohunt, 2018).

The exhaustion induced when navigating requirements and ingredients can lead to frustration and anger. In turn, this may lead to complaints when faced with yet another diet.

There is a lack of empathy brought about by exhaustion. It is understandable, but people with medically restricted diets end up being discriminated against, again. It isn't our fault that people are tired of too much choice. And it is hard to deal with when choice on a PKU restricted diet therapy is so limited.

Yet, we are faced with it in society and so need to find a way to handle such situations. I was put in such a situation not too long ago. One of my friends had been following the keto diet, and spoke of it enthusiastically when we met. It seemed that eating only protein had made them feel "just better, you know?"

I am practiced at trying to be sympathetic, and to ignore my inner voice screaming, when strangers or new acquaintances show a lack of tact when discussing diets. But this was my friend, someone who has known me for years. It made me think: "Wait, have they forgotten about PKU? Surely, they aren't trying to recommend this to me?"

After they listed the food they were eating, I replied that their current diet was essentially poison to me. There was an embarrassed silence which dragged on. Finally, I added: "Don't get me wrong, I would love to have that much protein. Especially after a heavy gym work out." My friend muttered something, and conversation moved on.

Why did I feel bad for reminding a friend about my PKU? Because I was pointing out their privilege. Being able to choose what you eat, or what you avoid, is not an option for anyone on a medically restricted diet therapy. But it was still a source of social embarrassment for both of us.

The prevalence of fad diets does mean that those of us with PKU will be having more interactions like the above. Or we'll be trying not to scream while someone complains about how hard it is to have to check all ingredients when shopping.

This is the downside of the fad diet phenomenon. For someone on a medically restricted diet, sitting through these conversations requires a big win to balance them out.

Taking the good with the bad

I'd argue that the trend towards plant-based and vegan diets does provide several marked benefits for those on the PKU restricted diet therapy. Let's start with the products available in those supermarkets.

I wasn't allowed cheese for the first 30 years of my life. But then coconut-based cheeses came out, and I was rolling in cheesy experiments. Toasted sandwiches, jacket potatoes, pizzas, & pasta all had cheese liberally added. I also came up with unusual combinations, and still enjoy banana and cheddar on toast.

There are many other products, of course. The development of oat, coconut, soya, and almond alternatives to milk has been a source of ridicule for some. But they mean that, for the first time, my family and I can have the same milk in our tea. This may not seem important, but small changes which help us feel less isolated do matter. Plus, the knowledge that you don't have to worry if you mix up the mugs while serving.

We celebrated this mild liberation in the hot drink department by buying a milk frother, which opened up a world of phe-free cappuccino and hot chocolate. The social media community are a good source to find out about more PKU-friendly products.

Eating out

There are further benefits to be found outside the supermarket. Eating out on any budget has also become much easier in the last few years. It used to be that there was only one dish on the average menu which might be tweaked for a lower-phe meal. In pubs, the meal was salad & chips, and the restaurant dish was some version of vegetarian risotto or pasta. "Hold the cheese, please".

The trend towards catering for other diets has been a boon. Obviously, the fact that a dish is plant-based or vegan doesn't mean that it is suitable for the restricted diet therapy. But there is more choice now.

The number of PKU-friendly dishes per menu has only increased slightly, but the variety has exploded. Once, in a single month before the pandemic, I managed to eat out on: both teriyaki and tempura versions of cauliflower; ratatouille tart tartan with vegan cheese; wild mushroom parmentier (a potato-based mash); and beetroot tartare. (Tartare is a usually raw steak, grated and served with a sauce. This substituted beetroot instead of meat so was PKU-friendly.)

More recently, the rise of plant-based meat substitutes has caused a problem for those navigating the PKU diet while eating out. Most of the meat substitutes (e.g., Beyond Meat burgers, seitan) are made from high-protein plants, or have added protein to supplement those on a plant-based diet.

These are appearing more often as the vegetarian option on a menu, reducing the choice for someone with PKU. I hope that jackfruit will resist this trend to remain a fixture on menus. I have written more about eating at home and outside the home in *Living with PKU*.

Eating at home

The restrictions of the pandemic months shifted my focus onto making inventive dishes at home. Weekends became a good time for experimenting and filling up the freezer with handy low-phe or phe-free meals.

Many of these were inspired, or permitted, by products available for those following vegan or vegetarian diets. Banana blossom took the place of fish in home-made, PKU-friendly 'Fish & Chips.' Banana blossom is another discovery helped by the trend to a plant-based diet. The flower of the banana tree is low in phe, and, once cooked, makes a decent substitute for fish.

Canned jackfruit became popular for its ability to mimic the texture of meat in vegetarian meals. Fortunately for us, it is phe-free, so becomes a useful addition to spaghetti bolognese or bbq burgers. Some of the recipes I followed were initially developed by PKU food companies, to showcase the use of their products for PKU. Most of the suggestions were recommended by others in the PKU community.

Additionally, I will often take a commercially available recipe and tweak it for PKU. Both banana blossom and jackfruit can be found in tins in large supermarkets or health food stores. I have written more about eating at home and outside the home in *Living with PKU*.

Recipes and ideas

The trend for alternative diets has produced new recipes. Some of these are not useful to someone on restricted protein intake. Others are great as a one-off, but are too difficult or time-consuming to make often. However, some new ideas are suitable for the daily PKU diet. A recent example is the Quorn 'fishless' fingers. This, along with sweet potato fries, provided my first 'fish finger supper'.

Note: This book does contain tips for meals, but it does not have recipes. These remain on my website at www.PigPen.page because the phe analysis of foods, and the recipes for commercial ingredients, are continually updated and the phe content of a recipe may often change.

18. Abnormal food behaviours and PKU

Managing a chronic condition affects every part of your life. When the management of that condition involves a food-based therapy, food becomes something of extreme importance. Not simply in a survivalist "find water, food, and shelter", way. Rather it is important because managing food is key to everyday life.

This links in to an obsession in many western societies with finding the "correct" type of food. For some people, food defines their entire lifestyle.

It is fine if someone willingly choses to follow a regime like 'paleo', and insist on sourcing "ancient grains". That is a choice they have made. A conscious decision to walk past the more widely available, and often cheaper, food stuffs to source the specialised food of their choice.

For someone with PKU, which is treated by restricting food, the choice is a starker one: Avoid 85% of all food stuffs, or risk brain damage. The choice may seem simple. But maintaining that course of action day after day, is exhausting. Exhaustion, and fear of what is on your plate, can lead to abnormal behaviours with food.

When you follow this reasoning, that conclusion should not come as a surprise to anyone. And yet, it came as a surprise to me.

It is only as I have grown older that I have realised my friends and family have a different attitude to foods than I do. When they go out to a restaurant, food is a major draw, a large part of the attraction and reward. For me, it is a hurdle to overcome so that I might socialise, and fit in.

My definition of a good restaurant is one which has a dish that will require a minimal amount of alteration before I can eat it. Insisting upon a restaurant with a dish that I want to eat, or one which I have been looking forward to, is setting the bar too high.

For PKU, a good restaurant is one with a dish which could possibly be changed to fit within a strict medical therapy with minimal disruption to the kitchen staff. There was one magical restaurant in Bruges where I was able to eat a starter, main, and dessert without any alteration. It wasn't a large or famous restaurant. But it has become a highlight of my life.

To reiterate: every day, we must treat our food as a potential threat rather than simply as an enjoyment. It is not a surprise that abnormal food behaviours are a feature of the PKU community.

I explained my struggle with diet anxiety earlier in this section. Over the years, I have learned to recognise when I'm anxious, and how to deal with those feelings in a way which doesn't affect my overall health. For a long time, I thought this anxiety meant that I was weaker than others. But, the opposite is true. Most people do not need to make a daily choice between food or brain damage.

Vomiting

Beyond anxiety over food, which can be debilitating enough, food behaviours can become terribly serious. Through-out my life, friends, and even new acquaintances have asked "can't you simply eat food and then throw it up later?" I have lost count of the number of times people have suggested this to me.

A close friend in high-school suffered from anorexia. Even so, other friends in the same group questioned why I didn't simply vomit up the food I wasn't allowed. Once I had outgrown school, other adults also proposed this harmful behaviour.

The suggestions were made by people trying to help me with an incredibly restrictive diet. But, they were still recommending a harmful practice. One which I avoided by talking to trusted family and friends.

When you ask someone for help, it can leave you feeling vulnerable. I understand the desire not to speak to a friend. We might need those around us to keep seeing us as they do. We do not feel able to speak to them, as it might change our relationship.

This is where counselling services can help. Having someone truly objective to speak with can be a gift. Often it is not until you say something out loud that you realise the power it holds over you. Then, you might begin to see the way through it.

Other mechanisms for coping with PKU may manifest as abnormal food behaviour. It is important for parents and caregivers to recognise that someone with PKU may not have all of these behaviours. But it will be a rare person on the PKU restricted diet treatment who does not have any.

Willingly eating non-PKU food

I initially titled this "sneaking food", but I am trying to be more careful with my language around PKU. Sneaking implies a furtive guilt. While that feeling may accompany the wilful eating of food which is harmful, there is enough guilt around PKU already.

In an earlier section, I described one of my indulgences in non-PKU-friendly food as a teenage rebellion. I wish this is all it was. Even as a middle-aged adult, I still find myself willingly taking non-PKU food from the cupboard. I am aware that this is not a good decision, yet I still do it. This means I hide my snacking. It is odd to say that as a grown adult. Who am I hiding it from? I do the weekly shop, I have full access to the kitchen, so who am I concealing my behaviour from?

It would be more accurate to say that, surrounded by the food of a household with non-PKU people in it, I simply run out of willpower.

It is so hard to avoid 85% of food. More so when the munchies (a desire to snack) arrive, and you are nearly out of the prescribed PKU foods, which aren't terribly satisfying anyway.

The reason many prescribed PKU foods aren't overly satisfying, is that they have no protein. Eating protein means you feel fuller. A meta-analysis which looked at the results of multiple research papers on this subject, found that eating foods with a higher amount of protein leads to greater sensations of fullness (Oaklander, 2016).

The munchies are a real and present danger for someone with PKU. Early in my career in the wine industry, I worked in manual roles which placed significant demands on the body. When your role requires heavy lifting and walking for 8 hours a day, lunch becomes both a serious business and a time for respite.

While my workmates would eat steaks, sausages, or have a proper bacon fry up before managing a 30minute snooze; I spent the entire hour eating plate-fulls of PKU pasta. There was simply no way to get the same kind of satiety in a short period of time. I have since learned that fibre also plays an important role in satiety, and there is more on that in *PKU and being Hangry*.

The avoidance of eating in public

There have been occasions when I have declined social invitations which involved eating in public. Typically, this happened when I was struggling with the restricted diet therapy, and knew that the temptations of an ordinary meal out with friends would be detrimental to my health.

The brain fog which comes with the higher levels of phe in the blood can make planning for eating out seem impossible. Brain fog also contributes to the difficulties involved with returning to, or regaining compliance with, PKU treatment. Not only is it a rigorous regime to establish, but someone struggling with the therapy may have an impairment in their decision-making. And, their willpower has been sapped just when they need to rely heavily upon it.

There have been other occasions where, while I went along with my friends, I did not join them for food. Either I would leave early, or make excuses to avoid the food. I did this because I was aware that if I did order anything, I would feel worse for it the next day.

It is not just the food which can cause this embarrassment and isolation. The PKU supplement is also a cause for anxiety when others are around. In the section on managing PKU, I discussed the need for a supplement to fit into your lifestyle.

Over the years, I had forgotten the school-yard teasing, which made fun of my "smelly medicine". Recently, I had a sharp reminder when meeting another person with PKU. Despite being into their third decade, this person was only just becoming with comfortable taking the supplement in the presence of others.

At school, they had hidden away in the toilets to conceal something which marked them out as different. Now, as an adult, they were just beginning to change that learned behaviour. They were building the courage not to hide this part of their medical treatment.

I was shocked and saddened to hear this. But I was not surprised. Nor could I judge them. The desire to fit in, and appear normal, extends beyond school. It is pervasive into adulthood.

On one occasion, my employer sent me on a training day. The fee for the course included lunch, and there was a request to email in advance with dietary requirements. I did so, using my handy email template (available in the chapter *Eating out with PKU*).

A few days before the event, I checked the planned buffet menu with the organiser. They were kind, and assured me that a plate of the acceptable hot dish would be set aside to ensure I would not go hungry. That part all went well, the dish was waiting for me and the kitchen staff were great.

However, during the introduction and registration session at the start of the day, the trainer asked who had made dietary requests and what they were. It felt rather inappropriate to reveal that to a room of strangers, indeed some of those strangers said as much to me later.

It was a simple training day, on a subject which had nothing to do with food or health. But right from the start, I was again marked out as different. While others networked over lunch, I was left to dine alone with my dietary requirements. I'm certain this was done politely; however, it was another disadvantage caused by the restricted diet therapy.

This is something which professionals who work with people with PKU have also noticed:

"I do see some who are less confident in some places, but it's difficult to be generalising on these things, as there is the potential of people having their energy sapped by the constant explaining (of) PKU to those outside the community." (McKeller, 2020)

When protein is the path of least resistance

For this reason, it can sometimes be easier to not discuss or explain PKU. My clinics and specialists have usually been happy with the status of my treatment. Some have even described me as a 'star patient.' However, there are times when I have resigned myself to eating non-PKU food because it is simply easier than the alternative.

In forty-plus years of living with PKU, excluding events organised for PKU, my sole social contact with another PKU person is a cousin of a friend of a friend who had a baby with PKU. Think of all of your friends over your lifetime, and then all of their friends, and then all of their extended family. One contact in forty years. That is how rare this is.

No-one has heard of PKU. Which means we have to explain it to everyone. This is exhausting, time-consuming, and in some cases, detrimental to our careers or social lives.

Is it any wonder that, occasionally, we might take the path of least resistance, and just eat what is on offer? Or we might skip the meal, choosing hunger over the need to explain ourselves again.

When put into the context of living with PKU, these differing behaviours around food are understandable coping mechanisms. But they are not normal.

19. PKU, depression, and fatigue

Depression is a term which is overused in our society. Missing out on a promotion may be disappointing or demoralising, but we will often use the word depressing instead.

Again, we need to be careful of our language here. While it is normal to be sad, or to feel low from time to time. It is not normal to always be sad or low.

Depression is a low mood that can last a long time, or keep returning, and it affects your everyday life (NHS website, 2022). Rather than an understandable reaction to difficult situations, like those described previously in this section., depression is a medically recognised, serious disorder.

Depression consistently interferes with daily life, and, in extremity, may lead to suicidal tendencies. If you are struggling with suicidal thoughts, it is important to tell someone you trust immediately. Most countries have a helpline which you can call for confidential help 24-hours a day.

Someone may become depressed due to their chronic condition. Because, however hard today was, your condition will still be there when you wake up tomorrow. The planning, and the anxiety, may crowd out happy thoughts.

PKU and its related treatments already have a marked effect on the daily life of those living with them. Emotional difficulties caused by managing PKU may also interfere. In addition, people with PKU may be predisposed towards depression due to the effect which high blood phe levels have in the brain. (See *What causes the symptoms of PKU?*.)

Fatigue

People with PKU need to know what we are having for dinner, before we can sit down to eat breakfast. This is necessary to ensure we don't exceed the allowed phe levels. There is no room for spontaneity with restricted diet therapy. A simple treat of a single biscuit with your morning tea, means you must completely rethink your lunch and dinner too.

Surveys by the NSPKU show that this planning takes about 20 hours per person per week. That is as much as a part-time job. A part-time job just to eat. And all that time could be spent earning income and contributing to society, or spending time with friends and family.

All this extra planning means that managing PKU can be exhausting, and depression can worsen this. Fatigue is a recognised medical symptom which goes beyond feeling tired. Everyone experiences tiredness, which is often alleviated by rest, or sleep. However, fatigue is when sleep and rest do not help with the tiredness (NHS website 2, 2022).

The constant tiredness which comes with fatigue can lead to low mood. Indeed, fatigue is one symptom of depression. This may sometimes turn into a vicious cycle of exhaustion, leading to low mood, which then leads to exhaustion.

Striving to stick to the PKU restricted diet therapy may take up the bulk of someone's capacity for thought. It will also take much of their willpower.

Willpower and PKU

One of the hardest things about PKU is that there is no cure at present. That it isn't following a food regime for a few months to lose weight, or to recover after illness.

When you get up every day, PKU is still there. There are new developments in PKU treatments (see *Beyond the restricted diet therapy*) which might help if available. But PKU is always there. That can be hard to accept. It is important to realise that acceptance is not resignation. Accepting that you have PKU is not resigning to the thought that treatments, and your life, will not improve.

Acceptance is not resignation

Accepting that PKU makes demands of you is not resigning yourself to the fact that it will never get better.

Accepting that you need to take more care over your food than normal is not resigning yourself to being abnormal.

Accepting that managing PKU is hard, (really hard!), is not resigning yourself to the fact that it is impossible.

Accepting that today was a difficult day (or week, or year) for you to manage your PKU is not resigning yourself to the fact that you will never be able to do so.

I realised this after a brain injury which was completely unrelated to PKU. After my injury, many parts of my life changed. There were things I could no longer do, and extra burdens of treatments to which I now needed to adjust.

I had to accept that things had changed. I didn't want change, and I certainly hadn't expected it. But now, change had been forced upon me. I fought hard to get to what I saw as a "normal way of life". It was exhausting. Sound familiar?

This was a particular feature of pandemic lockdowns. At a time when diaries were empty for months, reports of tiredness and mental exhaustion rose (Smith, 2020). When I called friends during that time, we'd all say "No, not been doing much. How about you?" Why did we feel like we were barely managing to get through the day?

Spoon theory

Initially, I didn't have an answer. But then, I discovered spoon theory. This is a metaphor to explain the reduced physical or mental energy available to someone with a disability.

This theory holds that our willpower comes in quantified amounts, e.g., spoonfuls. Each day we have a limited number of spoonfuls available. This means we must plan how to use our willpower, or we run out of spoonfuls.

This is similar to a theory by Professor Roy Baumeister, a psychologist. He explains that willpower is a type of energy. One which we should use wisely as energy levels can rise or fall. (BBC Bitesize website, 2022)

Spoon theory and PKU

Spoon theory illustrates the feeling of not having enough willpower to get ourselves out the door on a run when we have just finished hours of work. We've already spent all our spoons of willpower on just getting through the day.

When someone is living with a disability, or a brain injury, or a chronic condition like PKU, they are forced to spend spoons on simply managing that condition. This means they are disadvantaged when it comes to other daily tasks.

When you imagine your willpower as a limited number of spoons, you start to understand where all your energy goes. You may be drained, though it may feel like all you have done is prepare food. Spoon theory might help you to understand how much willpower is spent on living with PKU. It might also help you to decide on your priorities, where you want to spend your willpower.

Health, mental or physical, is an excellent priority. We will usually reap long-term rewards for the spoons of willpower spent on those priorities.

20. Community and support

I did not have a PKU community while growing up. Through a freak of history, New Zealand does not have many people with PKU.

As noted previously, the incidence of PKU varies across different genetic makeups. This book has used the incidence rate of 1:10,000, which is commonly accepted for populations of a European descent.

According to the 1 in 10,000 rule, the place where I grew up should have had about 400 people with PKU in the late 20th century. I was informed that there were only 120 of us in the country. The reason is obvious when you think about it.

Firstly, a substantial minority of New Zealanders are from ethnic groups other than European. In 2013, 75% of New Zealanders were from a European background, while 25% of the population come from ethnicities with a lower incidence of PKU. This is one reason why the 1 in 10,000 statistic did not hold (StatsNZ, 2019).

There is another reason, for which I do not have scientific backing. It stems from the fact that the European population of NZ derives mostly from emigration in the 1800s. Even though PKU was not diagnosed until the 1930s, it would still have been prevalent in the population at the time. However, it would have been completely unrecognised and untreated. Someone with the symptoms of untreated PKU would have been classed as mad & sickly. Many would have died young. Assuming they survived into adulthood, even a person with mild HPA is likely to have had some brain damage.

These are not traits which would be considered viable in an immigrant at the time; particularly not to an unknown wilderness on the other side of the world. In 1882 New Zealand brought in a parliamentary act to discourage immigrants who might place a health burden on the fledging colony. The Imbecile Passengers Act 1882 required a payment from all ships which might bring in someone considered to be lunatic, idiotic, deaf, dumb, blind or infirm.

Thus, I believe that New Zealand's relatively recent history of immigration has contributed to the low incidence rate of PKU in its European population.

Growing up without a PKU community

My first PKU event was in the UK before my family emigrated. I was young, not yet in school, and it was the NSPKU Christmas party. I remember a Santa Claus, and being special. Or rather, not being special. For once, I was the normal one in the room. One of the many children with PKU. My brother and sister, who did not have PKU, were the special ones for once. Even now, decades on, I can still remember this feeling.

Just as there were few people with PKU in NZ at the time, there were few PKU events. In my second year at university, I finally received word of a PKU event happening nearby. My flatmates all knew of my PKU, we lived and cooked together, and they accommodated the requirements as best they could.

They also approached the idea of a PKU event with a sense of fun, and came along to provide moral support. I spent a morning playing on the floor of a church hall with children who were all about 10 years younger than me. I was easily the oldest PKU person there, and at first felt like a square peg in a round hole.

We support those who support us

A lifetime of growing up differently prepared me for this, and I soon realised my presence was valued by the other attendees. Families, who had been coping on their own with the diet for years, now had proof that someone with PKU could thrive. I was someone who stood on the other side of the teen years and had made it to university. Living proof that there was hope in the struggle.

There was genuine relief that someone and their family had made it through the unique difficulties of teen years on the restricted diet therapy. In return, I learned of new PKU products which had made it to NZ, and new foods to seek in the supermarket.

This is the best reason to join a community of people with PKU: we learn from and support each other. Others in the PKU community have helped me to manage my own PKU. Their experiences have helped me to understand my feelings and struggles with the restricted diet therapy. Plus, few other people fully understand the joy when you find a delicious new phe-free food!

It can be hard to reach out, though. Every so often, the burdens of managing PKU among all the other struggles can just be too much. When that happens, we may need an added incentive, a bit of hope.

I have written about neuroplasticity in *Why do we manage PKU?*. This is the concept that the brain will respond to changes in our behaviour throughout our life. This concept is proof that we can change. Whether we are required to adapt to a small thing such as a new exercise routine or to something larger like building confidence to find others with PKU, our brains can do it.

Benefits from the PKU community

Of all the things I have learned from interacting with the PKU community, the most important lesson has been to listen. That might seem odd for someone who grew up being open, even overt, about their PKU. (And who has written a whole book about it.) However, not everyone's experience is the same. Everyone has a unique skill or struggle; we do have much to learn from each other.

Listening to others showed me that there is a need for an open discussion about the mental health challenges of PKU. There is a need for a wider awareness and discussion of the struggles which come with most aspects of PKU. This book came about with the help and encouragement of the PKU community. I encourage you to allow them to help you, too.

Participation brings a sense of purpose

Another good reason to participate is the mutual support from a community, which can bring clarity and purpose to living with PKU. You don't need to be everywhere, just chose a few ways to find a community which suits you. For years, I have participated in one small part of the social media world, and attended PKU events. The pandemic has reduced the availability of in-person events, and led me to further expand my online community. Social media has its faults, but it has proven a valuable tool in connecting people with rare diseases.

Over time, I have found a group of people who understand when I post about struggling with PKU supplements. People whom I can relate to, and support when they discuss problems. Several of these folks I would consider friends, despite never meeting them. In the past, we might have arranged to meet at a PKU event, but the pandemic has intervened there too.

A small interaction with others who are dealing with similar issues can provide a boost on a difficult day. Many of us will have come across that advice in the multitude of articles on caring for our mental health. Another tip is to find something which gives you a sense of purpose. That can be a little difficult to fit into an already hectic schedule, but we are talking a small change. Maybe taking 10 minutes once or twice a week to find people who are going through similar struggles.

There is scientific backing for the boost which participation can give to mood and mental health. During 2020, I discovered this for myself though a research study. This was a study into low mood following brain injury, but some lessons are applicable to PKU. The study was called MAPLES: Mood; Activity; Participation; Leisure; Engagement; Satisfaction.

The study was run by the Cognition and Brain Sciences Unit at Cambridge University. One of the goals in the study was to give participants tools to help increase engagement in activities which they find meaningful or enjoyable. At the same time, the team were looking at the difference between meeting as a group to plan individual activities versus meeting to participate in a group activity. The study had started before the pandemic, and was adapted to meet the new restrictions.

How activity affects mood

The course taught me about the links between activity and mood. This is a mood cycle whereby social isolation, like that experienced with PKU, can lead to a low mood.Someone experiencing a low mood might have lowered energy levels, which mean they avoid enjoyable activities, which then results in further social isolation.

This vicious cycle of isolation, low mood, low energy, and less activity feeds off itself, making each step worse in turn. This means it is easy to feel trapped in an ongoing cycle. But the good news is that a break in any one part of the cycle can lead to improvements elsewhere in the chain.

You might have already experienced this, where a bit of exercise can inspire you to meet someone, thus improving both your social isolation and your mood. Or you might go to a planned event, which lifts your mood, and you feel like exercising the next day.

This is known as behavioural activation. It means that the act of planning for an enjoyable activity, such as arranging to call a friend, can help us to feel less alone. This improvement in mood gives us more energy, which helps us to plan the next enjoyable activity.

I've noticed this myself after a walk, or workout, that my mood is lighter, and I feel ready to tackle new activities. However, even with the promise of a better feeling ahead, it can be difficult to drag yourself into an activity when in a low mood. This is where the PKU community and giving back through research participation has helped me.

How to kick out of the cycle

When we are in a low mood or have low energy, it can feel impossible to do more. Even if you know that you will feel better afterwards. This is where remembering to follow a plan, not a feeling, might help. This mantra works in several ways:

1. **A plan helps you to do something.**

Sitting around and waiting for your mood to improve rarely works. You need to do something about it. In difficult cases, that may mean talking to a counsellor or your GP.

2. A plan makes the decision for you.

You have talked yourself into doing something, what should that be? Rather than needing to spend more energy on a decision, a plan will have already made that decision for you.

Your plan might tell you that it is time to call a friend, or go for a walk. If you don't have a plan, then you can use that time to make one!

3. The next step is easier.

Once you have done something, you will usually have a bit more energy to try something else. This is a known effect where the motivation comes after the activity. That sounds odd, but how often have you found that doing one small thing on your list gives you a good feeling?

This is something to remember when managing or returning to the PKU restricted diet therapy. Changing one small thing might be all you can do at that time. But it is a change. And that can help to power your next small change. All these small changes do add up.

21. Tell someone that you have PKU

One small change which might have a positive effect is telling someone that you have PKU. Telling a person whom you often spend time with may make it easier to stick to the treatment.

This can be a significant step for some, as it involves trusting another person with information about you. This can lead you to feeling vulnerable, and vulnerable is scary. Talking about PKU can also be demanding; I've mentioned how exhausting it can be to continually explain PKU just to get through life.

In this instance, I mean to encourage you to talk to a person who you would like to understand your PKU. This might be someone close to you, yet who is unaware of your struggles. Or it might be someone more remote, but who might be able to make life a little easier; e.g., a work friend with whom you regularly lunch.

I've become more comfortable about describing my diet. PKU is a part of me. However, when I was younger, it wasn't fun to have to constantly explain PKU and my restricted diet therapy. No one wants to be different, especially teenagers.

Then I learned that life is easier if the people we hang round with know we were born with a medical condition. If they know that there is a serious reason why we are exacting about what we eat, and that the daily supplements really are medicine.

That may be as much as you want to tell others, or you might want to explain more. It is entirely up to you and how comfortable you are with the person you are speaking with.

But, telling someone you often see that you have PKU really can help.

Tips for talking to people about PKU

- Tell who you want, what you want. This is about making life easier for you. You don't need to explain yourself to others if you do not wish to.
- Don't feel you need to apologise. I try not to apologise for my PKU. Do you expect a diabetic to apologise for needing insulin, or when asking for low sugar alternatives? But equally, I don't expect people to have heard of PKU at all. It is a rare condition.

Talking about PKU can be easier if you have a few answers ready for **FAQs,**, like:

Does PKU mean we can't eat out?

Of course we can! We might need to be careful about where we go. A steak restaurant is not ideal, but roast veggies or salads can be found almost anywhere. Or, it may be possible to create a meal out of low-phe or phe-free side dishes.

I will order several sides and ask for these on a single plate as a main dish. Numerous places will offer side dishes like spring greens, or have sweet potato fries/wedges which are protein free. I have written more about this in *Eating out with PKU*.

Can I still cater for your PKU? Can you still come over to my place? Will you still come to my bbq?

Yes. This will be easier if many of your friends know about your PKU, but it is still possible if they don't. Many people are vegetarian these days, meaning that someone who hosts a bbq without a few veggies & salad is a bit odd. Ask if you can take something along for your main, like marinated aubergine steaks, or the low-phe halloumi substitutes which are now widely available. If you know that there will be food options for you, this can help reduce social anxiety, making for a more enjoyable occasion.

Do I have to explain my 'special' food?

You don't have to tell passing acquaintances about PKU. What you are eating or drinking is none of their business, you don't have to explain or apologise. Fortunately, comments on what people eat are becoming less common.

What do you eat for snacks?

Fruit is usually safe. For example, bananas & mandarins are phe-free, healthy, and already come in environmentally-friendly packaging. Plenty of breakfast bars are around that one-phe level. This is where we get to ignore the 'healthy' or 'ancient grain' labels and go for the chocolate ones; 'hey, is it my fault the double chocolate chip rice bars have less protein than some dry nutty monstrosities?

What about brunch?

If your friends or family are tucking into a fry up, perhaps you may join them with tomatoes, mushrooms, onion rings, and an exchange of beans or hash browns. Or, your friends might prefer to be healthy and have a smoothie.

Many places offer different smoothie recipes based on phe-free fruit, vegetables, juice, or coconut milk. (I've eaten apple crumble for brunch as it was the most attractive low protein option. Low protein is my priority, so I bend other meal-time rules to suit.)

There is no shame in asking for help

Even after living with PKU for forty years, I seek support and tips for my mental health. This does not mean I'm always struggling with anxiety or depression, rather that I am aware I need to regularly check on my mental state. PKU seems designed to trigger anxiety in a society with a complicated relationship to food. Where PKU is managed through the restricted diet therapy, this risk is amplified.

For many years, I muddled along, then a bad tackle during a football match gave me a mild traumatic brain injury. Initially diagnosed as a concussion, it took 15 months and many scans to determine that I'd had a bleed in the brain. This uncertain process triggered a mental health crisis. But, still, I resisted getting help. The stigma around seeking help for mental health problems is treacherous and ingrained.

It was only after three separate people, including health professionals, advised me to seek counselling that I did so. My only wish now is that I hadn't waited so long. Now I am open about the fact that I needed therapy. I encourage anyone who is struggling with their mental health to find someone, family, friend, or counsellor, to speak with.

One thing which might help is receiving answers to your questions about living with PKU. This is where the wider PKU community, whether online or in person, comes in. One adult with PKU spoke about this at a conference. She recalled the grandfather of a newly diagnosed baby, who pulled her to one side with a look of concern.

"Will my grandson ever just be able to have a pint with his mates?"

"Yes! He absolutely will. He'll need to count it because beer has alcohol, and he might have to be careful if they are also eating. But, yes. He absolutely will be able to just have a pint with his mates."

This is the kind of reassurance which only someone else who is living with PKU can provide. I urge you to seek similar support yourself.

Part five: Living with PKU

22. Planning with PKU

Once, while preparing for a brief presentation on PKU, I asked the online community: "If you had 200 words to tell a group of dieticians about living with PKU every day, what would you want to talk about?"

The answer was planning. Planning is a constant struggle for someone with PKU. It is a struggle, whether they are managing their treatment well, or not.

Every day must be planned around food. People with PKU are always thinking about food. Not necessarily because we enjoy food. But because we need to know what we are having for dinner before we sit down to breakfast. There is no room for spontaneity with restricted diet therapy. A treat of a single biscuit with morning tea means completely rethinking the phe allowances for all the other meals and snacks.

This means that it is rare for someone with PKU to be eating what they actually want to eat. It is not possible to eat on impulse. This book has laid out on numerous occasions the need to plan when living with PKU. So, what is the best way to plan?

Habits and routine

I have previously discussed how breaking a habit of buying the same foods can help with PKU. However, it is important to emphasise the critical role which habit and routines do have. A routine may be as simple as setting an alarm to take a supplement, or having them nearby when eating, so you can take them with a meal. A habit might be that of walking down, or avoiding, certain aisles of the supermarket to remember one food, or to avoid the temptation of another. Such habits and routines play a vital role in managing the restricted diet therapy.

Routine

Routines are everywhere at the moment. There are any number of search results for 'routines of successful people', or 'habits to set you up for success'. And some suggestions can help in managing chronic illness and conditions like PKU. But only if they work for you, as an individual.

Mark Wahlberg's routine is famous, and he is a successful actor. But I am not suggesting you get up at 3am to successfully manage your restricted diet therapy. Instead, focus on one easy thing to change. A habit which might help with your PKU, and an easy success which you can build on.

Breakfast is a good place to start. Not because of the proverb about it being the most important meal of the day. Rather, we usually eat breakfast at home, and might prepare it in advance. Both of these factors make breakfast a significant meal for someone with PKU. Starting the day with a diet-appropriate meal helps to set us up for success later in the day. And if the day becomes difficult, one where we must choose between a high-protein option or being hungry, at least there has already been one PKU-friendly meal that day.

Example: a PKU-friendly breakfast

A reader without PKU might not fully appreciate this emphasis on planning. Remember that planning for the restricted diet therapy is the equivalent to a part-time job. A survey of PKU patients in the UK revealed that planning for and managing the diet takes about 20 hours per person per week. Yes, there will be different levels of preparation and planning for those with a more restricted diet versus those who have more phe allowance. It is still more than someone without PKU might face.

I have attended PKU conferences with people whose phe allowance was only slightly higher than my own. However, it was enough to allow them to eat a normal continental breakfast from the hotel buffet. This is something beyond the scope of the more restricted diet therapies. Some with PKU will not be able to have commercially available cereal. Those of us with more severe PKU were restricted to the protein-free buffet of prescription bread, cereals, and 'milks' provided by specialist food companies. Even on tight or zero phe allowances, there are still options for breakfast, both with or without specialised medical foods.

One day, nearly a quarter of a century ago, a newly updated list of protein in foods informed me that I couldn't have cornflakes any more. New analysis showed that a 30g portion of cornflakes had 2.5 phe. A small bowl, even with PKU-friendly milk, would cost half of my 5 exchanges a day. It was simply not feasible to 'spend' that much phe on one meal. The news was devastating, and a good example of how far the phe-analysis has come in the past few decades. In the 90s it was still testing ordinary cereals, now the teams are reporting on more exotic items like mooli and samphire (both vegetables).

This letter told me, a teenager who just wanted to fit in, that breakfast was always going to be different. My Sunday's were spent diligently cooking for the week ahead. In rural NZ, neither bread-makers nor PKU specific cereals existed. For a few years, the answer was sweet corn fritters. While my (non-PKU) siblings were waking up, I was at the stove whipping up a double batch of fritters, hot ones for breakfast, cold ones for lunch. Bread making in the oven was not going well, so sandwiches were not an option in the lunch box.

It would be another decade until I discovered an easier solution to this breakfast puzzle. During work experience in the US, I came across a berry smoothie! They are everywhere now, but it was new at the time. My recipe has changed little over the years, and I still take five minutes in the evening to assemble it. Frozen berries, 10g (1phe) rolled oats and PKU-friendly milk or apple juice. This defrosts overnight, before I add a banana and blitz to a smooth consistency.

Preparing for failure

Sometimes life gets in the way, and we might be too tired, too busy, or too hungover, to follow our ideal plan. On those occasions, the mornings are a bit more difficult. Yes, I could defrost the berries in the microwave, but have you ever tried to drink a warm smoothie? Let's just say, it's not great.

At this point a dietician might be thinking, 'you have oats, just make porridge!' It comes back to managing the phe allowance. Those with more severe forms of PKU might only be permitted 5g of phe (or less) for the whole day. Ideally, this phe will be consumed with a supplement, and you are supposed to take your supplement at even intervals throughout the day. All of that means someone with PKU might have only 1 phe (or less!) available for breakfast. One phe (or 1 exchange) is 10g of oats. Even with sliced banana and raisins on top, that is enough for breakfast. And it must be made with PKU-friendly 'milk' or water.

Another alternative for breakfast is PKU-friendly toast, assuming it is available. Bread-makers are great, if you remember to use them. Ready-made PKU bread is convenient, assuming the delivery arrived. PKU conferences are also the only place where I have tried this type of bread. Despite the convenience, I haven't stopped making my own. I have owned a bread-maker since high school, and believe I was the first student at my university to receive a formal dispensation for a bread maker in a dorm room.

Bread makers have improved markedly since that time, and some have gluten-free cycles. This may be a better option when using the specialised PKU flour, which is often gluten-free. However, even a fast gluten-free cycle means waiting nearly three hours for a loaf. Rather too long to wait for breakfast.

As major supermarkets chains around the world expand their gluten-free ranges, some commercially available loaves may now be a convenient option for those with higher phe allowances. Some recipes come in at one phe per slice; however, there is still a need to find the exact brand. This means the early morning shuffle to a corner store for a loaf is still not an option for someone on the stricter PKU diets.

Back to cereal

What about PKU cereal? As someone who grew up without this option, I still consider a bowl of completely phe-free breakfast cereal to be a novelty. There are now several protein-free options available, either on prescription in the UK or for purchase in the US, Australia, and NZ. The same outlets also have phe-free milk substitutes available. At the same time, the societal shift towards plant-based diets means that many supermarkets carry plant-based milks, which can be lower in protein than dairy milks.

The expansion of plant-based diets has also led to a growing number of yogurt alternatives which may be suitable for those with PKU. These tend to be coconut-based, though caution is required as many recipes have higher elevated phe levels following the addition of soya protein.

Routine and habit may not replace the blissful normality of just sitting down and eating whatever you fancy at the breakfast table. But, having a routine and a few back-up options, make it easier to start the day with a PKU-friendly breakfast. This helps with managing the PKU diet over the rest of the day.

Tips for a routine

If you are new to PKU, or returning to the restricted diet therapy, or would like new ideas to spruce up your routine, here are a few suggestions.

Meal planner

It is important to spread the phe allowance out across the day, meaning it may be helpful to plan the daily meals in advance. This doesn't have to mean sitting down on a Sunday to write out a seven-day plan, though some people choose to do this.

During the week, there tends to be little variation in my breakfast or lunch (habit and routine!). So, I plan out my dinners for each day on a small magnetic chalkboard in the kitchen. This works for me because I enjoy cooking, and because I have a long-established habit of splitting my phe allowance across the day. If you are starting from scratch, then an extensive approach like planning all meals and snacks in advance might work for you. Or, you may decide to start with an easier habit.

Meal planning can be as simple as taking a moment each evening to think about the next day. For example, if you work outside the home, it might be helpful to get a breakfast ready and to measure out supplement the evening before. You might take a moment to think about lunch options. Adding a can of soup to your bag might provide a back-up option for lunch if there is nothing PKU-friendly at your office. You may not wish to think about dinner a full day in advance. But, when dinner time comes around, deciding what to have will be easier if you have already eaten a PKU-friendly lunch and breakfast.

A meal planner is whatever works best for you. You might prefer to do batch cooking at the weekend to fill up the freezer with convenient meals. Or you may prefer to avoid cooking, so it might be better to fill the freezer & cupboard with ready-meals, pasta sauces, & quick noodles which work for your phe-allowance.

Food diary

I wrote about food diaries in *Making PKU clinics work for you* because most people come across them through a request from a clinic. Because of this, a food diary can feel like homework. This sense of obligation may lead to resentment and guilt when completing them. But, a food diary can be a powerful tool to help manage PKU.

The key is to record what you are eating in a way that works for you. You might take a photo of your meals, or make a note on your phone. Or you may decide to use an app (see below). Keeping a food diary or recording what you eat, even if just for a few days, can be a worthwhile exercise. It is hard, nearly impossible, to manage or to change something when you don't know how things currently stand.

And that understanding may not necessarily be as bad as we fear. The human brain tends to focus on negative things, e.g., the meals which weren't PKU-friendly. We might remember these more than other, friendlier meals, and we might focus more on these perceived mistakes.

This means that, sometimes, our diet may be worse in our heads than it actually is. There is only one way to be sure, try out a food diary. Even if it never goes to a dietician, even if you are the only person who sees it, you will learn things about your PKU. And once you know something, you can choose to repeat it, or to change it.

Apps

There are now several apps designed to help with the management of PKU. Some are provided by companies which make products and supplements. Other apps, like the PKUCalculator, have been written by people with PKU specifically to help them with the restricted diet therapy.

Most apps have a calculator to assist with working out how much food is required for a certain number of exchanges. Some help you to track your phe and supplement consumption across the day. Others hold databases of foods to which you and others in the PKU community can contribute. With all these services in your pocket, an app can be invaluable for those who are:

- new to PKU,
- returning to diet,
- in need of help to work out the amount of protein in different foods,
- struggling with counting phe across the day,
- need reminders for blood tests or clinic appointments,
- or all of the above.

However, just because there is a service available, you don't have to use it. Some diet or recipe apps have meal planner functions, and cupboard integration. The idea is that, once it is set up, all meals can be planned for the week by adding recipes into menu slots. The app will then check its records of what is in the kitchen cupboards to produce a list of required groceries. This sounds fantastic, and I do have a recipe app with this function. However, I do not use it. The good old magnetic list on the fridge has always worked for me. Why fix what ain't broke?

Likewise, some PKU apps offer an option to record all blood phe results too. Again, this is a key attraction for some, while it may not work for others. We are already doing enough work managing the diet without having to worry about being on the cutting edge of technology. Use what works for you, and don't feel you are failing if you aren't using every service available.

Keep it simple

Staying on the restricted diet therapy can be exceptionally difficult. There are steps we can take which make it easier, such as having PKU-friendly foods to hand. Fruit is always a safe bet for a PKU-friendly snack. Bananas & mandarins are wonderful for trips away from home. They are phe-free, healthy, and come in biodegradable packaging which means they don't need washed before eating. Another option is bars, of the cereal/breakfast/muesli variety. Plenty of breakfast bars are around that one phe level. Some bars are now made with a marshmallow base, which makes them lower in phe.

Having PKU-friendly foods with us makes sticking with the treatment a little easier. It is also important for the mental and physical well-being of someone with PKU. Because, as discussed in the next chapter, we are often susceptible to hanger.

23. PKU and being Hangry

Hangry can be defined as being irritable or angry because of hunger. Hanger is another problem for those on the restricted diet therapy. Everyone gets hangry from time to time, but it seems to happen more frequently to me than to my friends or family. As a child, when my siblings and I were delegated to clear the table after dinner, I would always eat the remnants of the family-sized salad. No matter how much I'd eaten at the table, I could always empty the bowl.

Though I had eaten more than a full meal, and my stomach felt full, I didn't feel satisfied. My appetite never felt sated, and I often wanted to eat more despite the uncomfortable full feeling in my stomach. The phrase 'full stomach' never meant the same to me as it did to my siblings. Perhaps a stomach full of salad isn't as satisfying as one full of protein?

Spotting Hangry in the wild

I might be able to identify when others are hangry, but it can be difficult to spot in myself. In the past, I have dealt with this lack of insight through the diligent application of snacks. This was unconsciously done, but it became clear when my clinic asked for a food diary. My working days went something like this:

- 7am: home-made fruit smoothie with one phe, and a supplement;
- 9am: a bowl of PKU cereal with stewed apple on top (an actual second breakfast);
- 11am: PKU crackers topped with jam or honey for elevenses;

- 1pm: lunch, usually leftovers with one phe, and a supplement;
- 3pm: a biscuit or chocolate which might equate to one phe, and a supplement;
- 7pm: dinner of vegetables and PKU pasta with one phe, and the final supplement;
- 9pm: honey sandwich to ensure I didn't wake at night with hunger pangs.

In hindsight, I'm impressed the dietician didn't ask if I was part-hobbit. This food diary revealed that I was snacking at regular two hour intervals until 3 in the afternoon. There was then a longer break until dinner. It was in the early evening, ironically while making dinner, that I was frequently hangry. I'd heard several PKU people, both at conferences and online, discuss their need to eat regularly to maintain good levels of physical and mental energy. But this was a bit much.

Eat better, not more

After reading through this food diary, the dietician suggested I eat foods which would improve satiety. i.e., foods to help me to feel full for longer. They explained that if I could eat larger meals, less often (i.e., cut down on snacks); then I should find that my blood sugar remained stable. In turn, this should mean I avoided becoming hangry.

Those on the restricted diet therapy are supposed to spread out their phe allowance to coincide with meals and with their PKU supplement. Since I am allowed 5 phe exchanges and take 4 supplements, the new plan was to eat only four times a day. Breakfast, lunch, dinner and an afternoon snack to avoid hunger in the evening. This worked for me, but we are all different. What works for me may not work for someone else. But we don't know until we try.

Adding bulk to improve satiety

Psyllium husks: It was at a cooking demonstration for PKU that I first heard of psyllium husks. A professional chef hired by one of the specialist food companies discussed using it in PKU baking. Psyllium husks have the dual effect of assisting with the texture of the baking, and increasing the sensation of satiety (how full you feel) after eating the food. These husks are the outer coating of the seed of psyllium, a herb. They are used fairly widely as a source of fibre, and are often available in the larger supermarkets, high-street health stores, or online.

Psyllium husks are naturally phe-free, so allowed without counting on the restricted diet therapy. Plus, you need only a small amount in baking or for pancakes. It was the addition of psyllium husks which had the most beneficial effect on my satiety. I have always made my own bread, and adding husks to the bread-maker recipe meant I was now full after two slices of toast, rather than four. The texture was softer too, more like commercial non-PKU bread than anything I had managed before. Psyllium husks can also be used in cakes, muffins, scones, pancakes, waffles, and other baked goods to improve the texture. (There is more on baking in *Celebrations with PKU*.)

Rolled oats: This was another trick to add bulk and satiety to the food which I was already eating. I did this by adding rolled oats to my breakfast smoothie. I had first come across this idea while on holiday in Australia. Now, many places offer overnight oats, but that is not an option for someone on very low exchanges. However, the addition of one phe (10g) rolled oats to the morning smoothie helped me to feel more full after breakfast. When the pandemic meant I wasn't running out the door every morning, I began to eat the fruit and oats on PKU cereal rather than blitzed into a smoothie. This added to the bulk of my breakfast, and took me longer to eat, both of which increased the feeling of satiety.

What didn't work

There were many times when I wasn't organised. Perhaps I had a hangover, or there were too many meetings for a proper break. My most memorable working lunch was a coffee & a chocolate brownie snatched from the closest café. Not very PKU-friendly.

Life gets in the way, there are always reasons why I don't always follow my planned meals. But, time and time again, what didn't work was beating myself up over my mistakes. Or hiding from them.

Being kind to yourself may involve a little honesty. Honesty over why you did something, or avoided a situation. Honesty over whether your actions led to the best outcome. Perhaps even honesty with others over difficult situations and how they might help you with them. When we leave our home, we have less control over the situations and food which we come across, dealing with them can be simpler with a little planning.

24. Eating out with PKU

Eating outside the home is difficult to avoid, and can feel like a minefield for someone on a medically restricted diet therapy. I've written elsewhere (*Social Isolation with PKU*) about how the rise in the popularity of plant-based, and other, diets mean that menus can be easier to navigate, and staff have more experience in receiving diet-related requests.

It can be exhausting to steel oneself for 'that conversation' with waiters, or to hurriedly scan menus to see if we can eat at a particular venue. The thing is, people with PKU are worth the same service and attention as anyone else.

A little honesty about managing PKU in the real world

The dietary advice is to have the exact number of permitted phe exchanges, and to spread them evenly throughout the day. In a perfect world, this is how we would manage the PKU restricted diet therapy.

We do not live in a perfect world. The world in which we do live forces us to navigate the conflicting path between enjoying ourselves around food, and making the best choice for our health. In some circumstances, we need to make good decisions early, as these can then help us enjoy both our food and our social occasions.

Over time, I have learned that saving up one phe each weekday for a big blowout at the weekend is a bad decision. It comes back to that phenomenon where the symptoms of high-blood phe are quick to start, but can be slow to fade.

Often these mood disturbances, headaches, clumsiness, and tremors last for days, wiping out a whole week in return for one day of fun. It is truly not worth the damage to your brain. I strongly discourage this, though I understand how it happens.

We are also advised to spread the phe evenly throughout the day. If I'm going out that evening, yes I will make sure to have my normal breakfast and lunch with supplement, but I might save more of my phe exchanges for the evening. The next few days, I will have my exact phe allowance and take all the supplements. Yes, I know we aren't supposed to do this, and certainly don't do it every week! But, if the restricted diet therapy is getting in the way of you having fun, then you aren't likely to stick to treatment at all. It is about making the best choices you can in an imperfect world. Making those good choices becomes easier with support, practice, and confidence.

Confidence: because we're worth it

In a previous role, one of my colleagues was organising the office party and sent out the usual "any dietary requirements" question. I sent them my trusty template email (example pg. 156) which explained about PKU. In turn, my colleague sent these details on to the venue along with the other dietary requirements.

The venue responded with a request that I 'bring a lunch-box' as they were busy. My colleague replied that their response was not acceptable. If they wanted the company to use their catering, they would have to provide something for everyone. At first, I was shocked, then thrilled. This episode made me realise that, when eating out, everyone expects good service for their money; so why shouldn't someone with PKU?

It is common, and I know as I did it for years, to think: |the diet is my problem, so I'll just deal with it and not make a fuss'. But, actually most people are happy to help, if you have the confidence to just ask. Yes, you will need to be prepared for a few knocks. Refusal to help is increasingly rare in the world of social media and online reviews. Remember that in the rare event that you are refused, you can always look elsewhere. You do not have to give a venue your custom. I have found that the odd looks, and occasionally unexciting pasta-and-tomato dishes, have been far outweighed by fantastic experiences.

Remember: if you don't ask, you don't know what you might be missing out on! Confidence with eating out on the restricted diet therapy does grow over time. It will also improve as you become familiar with the treatment, and gain wider knowledge of what works for your PKU.

On several occasions, the service I've had has excelled that of my dining companions. There was a Michelin-starred chef who threw himself into the unusual challenge of catering for a PKU diet. (This was for a work function, I do not frequent Michelin-starred establishments.) Armed with the email I had sent through, this chef developed a PKU-friendly, 7-course degustation menu for me. I was in epicure heaven, while my companions looked on over their a-la-carte plates.

Another chef, this time in my home town, loved it when I came along as he could do something new. This was on the proviso that I booked with the restaurant at least a day in advance, so he could buy market-fresh produce just for me. That illustrates the next key to eating out:

Planning

If you can, it helps to contact venues and people before your event. Though this isn't always possible, we plan most celebrations or nights out at least a day or two in advance. Giving a venue notice of your requirements gives them time to adjust dishes and find ingredients. If you have contacted them before they purchase food, your requirements will be in mind as they buy.

If you have a significant event coming up, perhaps a holiday or a wedding, contact the venue and see if they can help. Try to avoid calling a restaurant during service hours, which are usually 11:30-2pm and then 5-11pm in anglo-centric countries. This is because working kitchens are busy places. Staff will have more time for your request if they are not having to juggle other guest requirements.

For this reason, I will often send an email instead. It gives the reader time to absorb the information without putting them on the spot for an answer. If you prepare, and can provide clear information and guidance, you may be amazed at what happens.

Included below is an example of the template email which I send to hotels, restaurants, conferences, wedding venues, & etc. Be sure to ask your PKU clinic or dietician for help in adjusting it to your requirements before using it.

Replacing the trial of having to explain about your "'special diet" into the smooth assurance that "chef has prepared a special menu for you" is a joy I cannot tire of. A little pre-planning with restaurants can turn the worry of a night out into just enjoying a great night out.

Example email

One of our party is on a medical, low protein diet. The restrictions are no meat, fish, shellfish, bread, tofu, legumes (e.g., chickpeas, lentils), nor soya. They are not allowed eggs, though the small amount in pasta is allowed. Dairy products are restricted, though again the small amounts of butter and cream in sauces are fine, as are meat-based stocks. Most vegetables and fruits are also permitted.

Usually, the easiest option is a slight tweak to an existing pasta, or rice-based vegetarian dish; though this cannot have cheese. Do you have a sample menu which might help with this request? Please do let me know if you feel I can be accommodated. I am happy to speak to a member of your team about this, or about adapting some of your current dishes. Do let me know a convenient time to call.

Note: this is an example for someone on a severely restricted diet. You will need to tailor it to your requirements and permitted foods. I always include the word 'medical' to ensure the reader knows that I am not simply being picky or trying out a fad diet. Remember, if you are booked in as a member of a larger party, you have a little more weight to throw around. If you are looking locally, you may wish to say you are looking for a great local restaurant for regular meals. The incentive of return custom is always attractive to venues.

Tips when eating out spontaneously, or for low-key occasions

The planning set out above is less useful if you haven't had a chance to call ahead, or if you are out on a lunch break, or with friends. In these situations, families, groups, and social media can prove invaluable.

Eating out as a family or group

Meals when eating out or on family holidays tend to revolve around the restricted diet therapy. This was certainly my experience when growing up. Eating out as a family was a good training ground for managing my restrictions when eating out later. This also helped me to manage PKU when I left home for the first time. It was with the support of my family that I learned to navigate a menu, looking for PKU-friendly dishes or those which the kitchen might easily adapt.

This may sound difficult, but it does get easier over time. There were five in my immediate family, which meant deciding what to order was a communal affair. "Would you like to share some sweet and sour noodles in return for the broccoli which comes with your chicken?"

In my memories, this light bartering of dish components to meet PKU restrictions ran smoothly. Recently, though, my mother revealed that she would always wait until everyone else had ordered. If there was enough for me to eat, then she would be able to order her first choice. If the conversation hadn't been able to source a full dinner for me, then she would order her back up. And we always ordered extra salad for the table. Everyone knew I would eat the lion's share, but it was always ordered for the table to avoid singling me out. These are a few small tricks which we used to make things as easier when dining out.

A family might eat out for breakfast or brunch as an indulgence, or when on holiday. Those with PKU can have a fry-up of phe-free tomatoes, mushrooms, onion rings; perhaps with PKU-friendly 'sausages', beans, hash browns as the phe allowance. I like making waffles at home, and will often 'spend' most of my daily phe on waffles when eating out. (See point above about living in the real world.)

Yes, there has been the odd disappointing meal, or repetitions of 'salad & chips'. Being able to share dishes with family and friends helped to alleviate otherwise difficult meals. And as I become more comfortable with phe-free and low-phe options, with portion sizes, and with discretely taking a supplement, eating out became easier.

In my life, I've emigrated twice with PKU and taken my dietary restrictions & supplement to over 15 countries. This has meant asking a variety of chefs to cater for a PKU diet. Even the meat-loving, cheese-adoring staff in a restaurant in the heart of France were accommodating (after looking at me as if I was from outer-space).

Look online

This is another area where a PKU community can help. We might grow connections by meeting others with PKU at social events. Or, as has become more common, interacting online. I often see a request for help with somewhere PKU-friendly for a special occasion, or when visiting a new city. The best source of PKU-friendly places is others with PKU.

If you don't have a community which can help, then a quick online search can be useful. This is another area where the rise of plant-based and vegan diets has helped those of us living with PKU. As the prevalence of meat-free dishes has grown, so too has the advertising and ease of finding such places. There are now websites dedicated to restaurants and cafés which serve vegetarian, vegan, and plant-based dishes. However, given the varying needs of different PKU requirements, we still need to check each menu carefully. As hospitality venues upload more sample or current menus, this task becomes easier.

Don't overlook the possibility of discovering an exciting place to eat through a quick search. Wiki-travel listings of vegetarian restaurants helped me find a venue in Bruges, Belgium. Vegetarian restaurants do not automatically work for the restricted diet therapy. However, I was able to order the three-course set-piece dinner straight off the menu without having to change anything!

The last tip here, is to have a backup. Being adventurous with our trips and meals out is great: again, it is easier with a little preparation. It can be particularly helpful to avoid decisions made in hanger. Therefore, having a banana or a supply of PKU biscuits in the bag is a must for days out in strange places.

25. Travel & emigrating with PKU

Travelling with PKU is definitely possible. Like anything, it does involve planning. But, it can still be exciting and spontaneous. A few years back, before the pandemic, I planned a staycation. There were things which needed to be done, and I figured taking a week to sort them would make life easier.

I finished those tasks in a day. Rather than kicking my heels, I spent the rest of the week on a spontaneous road trip round Ireland with a few friends.

My PKU requirements for the trip fitted into a backpack, along with all my clothes & everything else. Despite the supplements, mixers, and food, I was not the person with the largest luggage in our group.

In my bag I had sachets of the supplement needed for each planned day, plus two days spare just in case. These were packed in with a letter from my dietician explaining their function. I always travel with these letters, in case customs ever have questions.

My backpack also contained PKU biscuits for snacks, a few packs of individually packaged PKU bread rolls, and a ready mix Mac & Cheese pot. I had picked these up at a PKU conference earlier in the year, and held on to them for just such an occasion. It is possible to be spontaneous with PKU. Ironically, it is easier with preparation.

Sticking to the diet vs having a break

The temptation to reward yourself with time off from the restrictions can be considerable. A holiday is a break from everything else, why can't it be a break from PKU too? There are several important arguments against going off diet for a holiday treat. What may seem like a treat can interfere with the other benefits which a holiday brings.

It is difficult to relax when the anxiety from high blood phe levels hits hard. And the effects of high blood phe levels can start early in a holiday. A holiday is supposed to be a happy, relaxed time. A protein headache, and its effects on mood, planning skills, and energy levels, can reverse those feelings quickly. It is possible to have a great holiday, complete with treats, and stay on PKU treatment too.

When I started travelling with PKU, I'd pack everything I might ever need; with a special emphasis on snacks. It seems a common trait that people on the restricted diet therapy have an anxiety about going hungry. The truth is, a banana and a bottle of water can be bought easily in most holiday destinations round the world.

Longer trips

If you are going for longer than a few days, some PKU medical supply companies can arrange for your food & supplement to be delivered to your accommodation, within reason. In the UK, this tends to mean Europe, and the service is handled through the home delivery services.

When I visit friends and family in New Zealand, it is always a longer trip. And my home delivery company cannot arrange for my supplement and prescribed foods to be sent. The last time I flew, all of my supplement for three weeks, plus several extra days in case of emergency, was split between my carry-on and checked luggage. I recommend you split your food & supplement if you can't carry it all on, just in case a suitcase goes missing.

The option to carry on your supplement is trickier if you take a ready-to-drink supplement rather than powder or tablet. But I have put PKU supplement into baggage hold too, and never had problems. Though always ensure they are packed in with letters, should customs become curious. If you are putting liquid supplement in the baggage hold, do not stint on plastic bags. Ensure they are well wrapped, and away from anything which may pierce them!

Dietician letters

The first clinic letter which I remember carrying was for the trip to Japan as a high-school student. My dieticians detailed the types of supplement and prescribed foods which I carried, and explained that these were to be treated as medicine. I took a copy to my school teacher, who translated it into Japanese.

When I first reported at check-in, there were copies of both translations of this letter everywhere. They were in my hand, in my backpack with the carry on supplement, plastered over and inside each box of the supplement going into the hold, and in the hands of all adults who were chaperoning the trip.

To date, I have carried letters explaining my supplement and prescribed foods from the UK to NZ, and back again; as well as to island nations in the Pacific Ocean, into the USA, Japan, China, & all over Europe. It was only recently, in Australia, that a customs officer ever asked to see it.

My career started off with working in wineries and vineyards in New Zealand and the US. The stint in the US was a 4-month contract at a winery for their vintage, or grape harvest. As with the trip to Japan, I carried my supplement, Maxamum

XP, with me. I can tell you that reporting to US customs with 40 kilograms of a white powder in my suitcases was an interesting experience! I was clutching the letters with white knuckles in that queue.

But I wasn't even stopped and was waved through without a problem. That was three weeks before the attacks in September 2001. On the way back to NZ, three months after that terrible day, I was stopped for the nail scissors in my hand luggage. Again, there were no questions about the supplement or PKU foods. However, I would always advise taking dieticians letters with you when travelling, why tempt fate?

Supplement while travelling

Taking supplement while travelling can be difficult, the key is to stick to your routine and consider it to be a part of your meal. While I do know of some people who check out immediately after breakfast, I've always headed back up to my hotel room before checking out. This gives me a chance to take the morning supplement, brush my teeth, and clean the shaker, so it is ready for the next dose. A clean shaker is one less barrier to taking a supplement while sightseeing.

I do take my supplement, even when struggling through football tournaments in 30 degree heat with massive hangovers. I may not always take it at the ideal time, and have sometimes ended a day taking two supplements at once before crawling into bed. However, my holidays, and hangovers, are always better for doing so.

The supplement which works for you in everyday life may be the most suitable for travelling. Or it may not. A holiday at an-all-expenses-paid resort is different to one spent sightseeing and with new accommodation every day. Just as samples of

PKU foods can be handy for a holiday, this may be a good time to try a new type of supplement.

Perhaps a trial pack of tablets or micro tabs would be a good fit for a holiday with lots of accommodation changes? Or you may feel that sticking to supplements is hard enough without any changes. In this instance, have a think about how taking a supplement might be easier for you. That might be taking a supplement first thing, so it doesn't interfere with breakfast. Or taking it last thing at night once rich dinners have settled.

Routines slip when we are on holiday, it is part of taking a break. But we also go on holiday for rest and happiness. High levels of blood phe can interfere with this, so do try to have the supplements if you can.

Eating and drinking while travelling

Eating in a new country can feel daunting; just like anything with PKU, a little planning goes a long way. If your holiday will be self-catering, this may be easier. Even if you are flying overseas, it is possible to take PKU supplement and prescribed foods with you. If you are already signed up to receive your prescriptions delivered directly to your home, some of these services offer delivery to holiday destinations in the UK and some overseas destinations too. Or supplement may be packed in hold luggage or as carry-on, though be careful with the rules on liquids.

If not, and as I noted above, it is possible to take PKU prescribed foods with you. Some airlines allow extra baggage allowance for medicines, check with the company you are booked with. The types of specialised food which you take may be dependent on the type of accommodation you have planned. Taking a box of pasta to a large hotel may not work, and you may prefer not to explain PKU to a large kitchen staff. Some B&B owners have been receptive to toasting PKU bread for me, once I have assured them that I do not have an allergy. Even the basic catering of a tea and coffee area can work. There are PKU food companies which supply pasta pots, where all you need is a kettle for a hot PKU meal.

Whether you self-cater or not, most holidays will involve eating out. However, breakfast is usually in the place where you are staying. This is the first opportunity to set your PKU up for the day. Whether travelling for business or fun, with people or without, taking something phe-free for your breakfast is a good move.

My breakfast at home tends to be a smoothie, but I will often pack the prescribed PKU breakfast cereal into a suitcase. Most hotels are perfectly happy for you to take your own cereal and fruit from the buffet. I have found that some PKU cereals are sweet enough to take with water or apple juice, which is easily found at breakfast tables. It is also good to have one phe-free meal to count on in the day.

I have travelled on huge organised trips to sports tournaments in several countries, including meat-focussed places like Czechia (Czech Republic) and Bulgaria. Naturally, these tournaments were to test the limits of our physical ability, especially since the beer was free. Prague was a challenge, being the land of the pork knuckle. The vegetarian option at one venue was the horse-radish sauce.

However, I had alerted the tour organisers to the requirements of a restricted diet therapy in advance, and they prepared a meal for me. It isn't fun having to ask and being singled out. But my team-mates already knew about PKU, and they wouldn't let the staff rest until I had eaten enough. The beauty of letting people know about your PKU is that they can support you.

I first discovered this during that trip to Japan. There were sixteen of us on the trip, though this was high-school, so there were people I didn't particularly want to explain PKU to. I did make brand-new friends on that trip, people who I had never imagined would be kind to the person who they had often dismissed as "picky about food". Once they saw that I had to be careful even on the trip of a lifetime, they realised that it wasn't something I was doing for the attention. They stopped teasing me and, when we returned to school, stopped others from doing so too.

Actually, with many of us away from home for the first time and missing home comforts, meal times became an exercise in bargaining and negotiation. For example: "The beef is good, and currently the highest bid for my slice is from Susie. She offers all her vegetables and half the ice cream, do I have any advances on that?"

My school friends were also keen to help out with mixing the supplement while travelling. In heavy turbulence over the Sea of Japan, it took seven of us to successfully measure and mix the powder and water to a potable substance. All part of the adventure, and it taught me that usually people are happy to help, if you only have the confidence to ask. This can take time and practice to acquire, and many of the tips in *Eating out with PKU* apply to travelling too.

As an adult, I travelled regularly for leisure and business, before the pandemic put an end to such things. One trip for my employer involved ten days in Japan researching the sake production process. By the end of that visit, I was a demon at eating salad with chopsticks.

Managing PKU proved even easier on my return to the land of the rising sun. Having the supplement in a sachet form, rather than in 500g tubs, is far easier to pack. It is also much easier to mix and use when out and about during the day.

Once again, I took the breakfast cereal with me, along with some PKU biscuits for emergencies. It is always good to be able to snack without needing to count the exchanges. I had sent on my trusty example email in advance, and the catering on the trip was outstanding.

One place which hosted us had prepared a 20-course Japanese banquet matched to different sakes. The team had also prepared a special 20-course PKU-friendly Japanese banquet just for me. It was a wonderful experience.

There is, however, always a challenge in life. I am still trying to find the best aeroplane meal for a PKU diet. At present, I think Asian vegetarian is the lunch or dinner option to go for. A version of a vegetable curry is a fairly solid bet. It comes with rice, which works well for those needing to fulfil a phe exchange allowance, though any paneer for tofu in the dish should be avoided. However, the breakfast option on flights is still a challenge.

Tips for PKU travel:

- Take extra supplement for emergencies;
- If supplement isn't in your carry-on, split it between several bags in the hold;
- Find out about the meal options on any flights;
- Think about the snacks you might find locally, e.g., fruit and vegetable availability;
- Take a phe-free breakfast option;
- Spend a bit of time thinking about the catering services at your accommodation;
- Look online for vegetarian or vegan friendly places, as these are more likely to be able to cater to PKU restricted therapies.

Emigrating with PKU

Moving to a new country, and gap years, are a part of normal life for many people. And they are certainly possible for those of us with PKU.

You may be sick of reading the word 'planning' by now, but this is another area where it can help. I first moved halfway around the world in the mid-80s. This was before the internet made finding information and contacts as easy as it is today.

My next big move was to back to the UK, in 2005. I had a final appointment with my PKU clinic just before leaving NZ. This gave me confidence that my diet was on track. Due to the links between the UK and NZ health systems, my NZ clinicians could advise on signing up with the NHS. I had UK citizenship, which helped with this.

Our initial plan was to stay with my grandparents, and I posted supplement and prescribed foods to them in advance. This is a great idea if you have an address before travelling. I carried more in our suitcases, and my parents were on stand-by to post extra. This helped in the first few months while I was setting up a new home.

As soon as I had a home with proof of address, I headed to the local doctor to get signed on as a patient. The aim was to sign up for supplement and foods. I had moved a few times within NZ, so already had experience with signing up to new doctors.

While you may come across a doctor with prior experience of someone with PKU, that is a rare occurrence. Do not be alarmed by this, PKU is uncommon.

In most cases, you will have to explain what you require from the doctor to help you live with PKU. Preparing for this, and taking notes and someone for moral support, may be useful. The NSPKU have information sheets for doctors and for other medical staff. A key tip would be to remain clear on what you need:

- Access to prescribed medicines, including specialist medical food items which are not available anywhere else.
- A referral to the local PKU clinic.

26. Celebrations with PKU

Celebrations, an occasion for joy, can be difficult for people with PKU. What steps can we take to ease our difficulties and make celebrations more enjoyable? A little knowledge can go a long way, so here are a few things I've learned across the years.

Cold days

Language is important when it comes to PKU and food. The term 'Sunday roast' has come to encompass a social gathering, a weekly family ritual. It is also a term which may cause someone on PKU treatment to feel left out.

Simply putting a little thought and preparation into catering for someone on the restricted diet therapy will go a long way to combating their anxiety and isolation. For those of us with PKU, it can help to focus on dishes besides the main one; I rarely come across people who only have meat in the oven. Depending on how restricted the diet therapy is, common roast vegetables which are low-phe include: parsnips, carrots, sweet potatoes, turnips, swede, and sprouts.

Obviously, as I grew up in NZ, my family tucked into lamb. However, there was still an emphasis on catering for PKU. So, in our house, it was always "the PKU dinner and the roast". I believe I have tried every form of stuffed vegetable possible; squash is always a good bet. Stuffed capsicums (sweet peppers) are easier to prepare. Watch out with courgettes, as they tend to be wet.

In the last few years, some low-phe pastries have appeared. I've used them to make butternut squash & sage wellington with blue 'cheese'. This utilised a vegan blue cheese substitute which was low enough in protein for inclusion in my diet. I have also used this pastry to adapt many 'normal' recipes, including for individual jackfruit & portobello mushroom wellingtons which make a good PKU centrepiece for a celebration. The pastry has also proved its worth in caramelised onion and (PKU-friendly) feta tarts, as well as in apple strudel. (Recipes on www.pigpen.page)

Warm days

A childhood spent in NZ meant sausage sizzles (a bbq focused on hot dogs) and other bbq's. Sausage sizzles were difficult, but not impossible. My mum and I would spend wet weekend days stocking the freezer with 'sausages' to ensure a ready stock for bbqs. These 'sausages' were made from cooked, mashed protein-free vegetables which were then rolled in PKU breadcrumbs. We also made burger patties in the same way.

Now, several of the companies who make specialist food products also make a mix which fulfils this role. This mix allows someone to make a PKU-friendly burger or sausage and throw it on the bbq, or into the frying pan, in less than a minute.

That wasn't available in my childhood, so we had a different back-up plan. If we didn't have time to defrost 'sausages', or had run out, then aubergine (eggplant) worked well. Cut into rounds, marinated in some Tupperware on the way to the venue, these 'aubergine burgers' were also a bbq staple.

Recently, with the increased prevalence of plant-based, vegetarian, and vegan diets, I am spared the need to make mashed versions of sausages. There are now plant-based sausages in major supermarket, though some contain high protein as a feature intended to endear them to vegetarians. Some of those sausages derived from soy and pea protein are still low enough in protein to be available to those on higher phe allowances.

Those of us on lower phe allowances need to look at those foods derived from phe-free vegetables like mushrooms or jackfruit. There are also vegan versions of 'halloumi' derived from coconut oil, which may also be a good bbq option for someone on the low-protein restricted diet. Do note that these tend to work best on the flat plate side of a bbq, rather than the grill side.

Away from the hot foods, most bbq hosts will offer a plentiful selection of fresh fruit and vegetables in the form of salads. It was only when I came to the UK that I came across widespread use of cheese and/or bacon in salads. This proved problematic, until I learned to ask for 'green salad', and most people do provide a version of a green salad when hosting.

The informal setting of a bbq can make it easier to avoid odd looks or questions from others about what you are eating. If you are nervous, then please remember that you don't owe anyone an explanation for what you eat.

Cakes and birthday parties

I love cake and have a sweet tooth. I also happen to enjoy baking and have included some tips on PKU baking below for those interested. However, if you are not a baker, there are still plenty of options for PKU-friendly party cakes and snacks.

At the time of writing, at least one of the specialist food providers in the UK were offering a baked-to-order PKU cake service. This service was limited to a geographical area due to the nature of the fresh product. I was unable to find similar services elsewhere in the UK or other countries. However, I hope for an increase in businesses offering services for PKU and other restricted diets.

There are PKU cakes available, either on prescription or for purchase, from companies which provide specialist food products. However, most of these are single-serve cakes. This makes sense, as they are easy to carry and to serve as a handy PKU snack. But, it means such cakes are not suitable as the centrepiece for a birthday or celebration.

The same companies do offer alternatives which work well for a low protein birthday or celebration cake, though they involve a small amount of effort. Several companies offer PKU-friendly cake mixes. These all require the addition of wet ingredients, usually water or PKU-friendly milk, before being mixed and then baked.

These cakes can be decorated, just as any other cake might be. The days of needing to mix up icing sugar and food colouring have gone, though you can still do this if you wish. There are many icings and cake decorations available in stores which are low in protein. Many of the resources provided by patient organisations will have lists of those available in your area.

It is possible to have a PKU-friendly cake as the centrepiece of your child's (or child-at-heart's) birthday party. If you would like to serve non-PKU cake to the other children and save as much of the PKU cake for your child later, there is a trick which might help.

Buy or make a non-PKU cake which is similar to the PKU cake, and with the same icing. After presenting the decorated PKU cake for the candles and song, take the cake back to the kitchen to cut. In the kitchen, you can cut both cakes and plate them up for service to the PKU and non-PKU children as appropriate.

This does involve a little diversion and distraction on the day, but it does work. Apparently, my mother did this for parties right through my childhood. I had no idea until she told me once I had grown up. If you feel a little bad about it, it might help to consider it as a magic trick. All magic is about diversion and sleight of hand.

This trick of serving slices of similar cake directly from the kitchen can help if your child has PKU and is invited to a party where the cake will not be PKU-friendly. If you can ask beforehand for the colour of the sponge and icing, a similar cake can be made in an evening from PKU cake mix and decorations.

Baking with PKU

My skills at baking with PKU flour and egg replacers has improved over the years; particularly with the addition of psyllium husks. If you also bake, most specialist food supply companies provide recipes for their products, and the PKU online community also shares recipes and tips. (My recipes and tips are on www.pigpen.page)

My main advice for baking with PKU flour would be to think gluten-free. Frequently, the flour manufactured for PKU is also intended for gluten-free needs. This means it can benefit from some of the same steps used in gluten-free baking. These include:

Heat

One of the pioneer gluten-free bakeries in London recommended ensuring your oven is hot when baking with gluten-free flour. This is because gluten forms a large part of the structure which holds up the rise in baked foods. As this is missing in gluten-free baking, the mix will not maintain the rise from the yeast, baking powder, or baking soda for long.

This means you need to ensure your oven is at the correct temperature when the baking goes in. I discovered how important this is when my baking magically improved after moving house. The oven in my old flat had tended to be too cold, though I didn't know it. This meant that the time between mixing the wet & dry ingredients, which activates the rise, and getting the cake mixture to the correct heat, was too long.

Now, I will wait for the oven to reach temperature, sometimes waiting to mix the wet and dry ingredients until I know the oven is hot, or even 5 degrees over temperature. Then I will mix the wet and dry ingredients together, which activates the rising process. The trick then is to quickly get the baking into the hot oven.

Psyllium husks

The chapter *PKU and being Hangry* discussed the effect which the addition of these phe-free seed husks have made to my satiety (or how full I feel after eating). These husks can be used in cakes, muffins, scones, pancakes, waffles, and other baked goods to improve their texture and help those with PKU to feel fuller after eating them.

They help with the creation of a structure to hold the rise in the mixture. Combined with the correct heat setting (see tip above) these two small changes can have a marked effect on PKU baking. Psyllium husks are widely available in the larger supermarkets, in health stores, or online.

Fats

This tip comes from a cooking demonstration held by one of the chefs employed specifically to work with the medicated foods from specialist supply companies. The lack of gluten in the flour means that, in some cases, the flour will benefit from being coated with the fat (the butter, shortening, lard, oil, etc.) before you get on with the rest of the recipe. That needn't be laborious; it is essentially the same as rubbing butter into flour, which is called for when making pastry or crumble.

Coating the flour with the fat seems to help with the 'thirsty flour' phenomenon. This is not a scientific term. Rather, it is one I came up with to describe the ability of PKU-specific flour to soak up more water than the recipe calls for. Time after time, I would mix the wet & dry ingredients to the required texture and start doling out cookies, only to find that the mix continued to dry out. The dough seemed to continue to absorb the water while I was working. Applying this tip of mixing in the fat to the flour first seemed to reduce this phenomenon, and resulted in a cake which was more moist.

I am a baker, but a lazy baker. Rather than carefully rubbing cubed butter into flour with cool fingertips, I put it all in a food processor and whizz it. This is also a good time to ensure that any dry seasonings (like powdered ginger or cinnamon) are distributed evenly in the mix.

Patience

This tip is not related to the gluten content of the flour, but it is a necessary and oft neglected ingredient when baking. Taking a little more care in mixing, measuring, or with baking trays & tins can make or break the result. This also holds once the baking has come out of the oven. Leaving baked goods to cool properly before decorating or cutting can lead to a marked improvement in its appearance, texture, and longevity.

PKU at Christmas

Christmas is not the only event which is commemorated annually, usually as a family gathering. However, this is a book about how I have lived with PKU over the last decades. Sadly, I have little-to-no experience of Thanksgiving, Eid, Seder, or other ritual events in which food or fasting feature. I hope to include sections on these celebrations in future editions.

Christmas food

Christmas is a time when food tends to be everywhere, and different families have different celebrations. In NZ, Christmas was in the middle of summer. Our Christmas Day always started with a swim followed by brunch on the patio. My family would have smoked-salmon-on-toast. My special treat was semi-dried tomatoes, I'm a child of the 80s. In the week before Christmas, my parents ensured that I was involved in the purchase of the bright red tomatoes from the local speciality deli. It was a special occasion beforehand, as well as ensuring I had phe-free treats on the day. This was important as I could gorge myself on some foods without me, or my parents, worrying. Other phe-free treats were fresh exotic fruit like melons, papaya, & mango.

My parents had a rule that my siblings and I were allowed to open our stockings when we woke up. But we weren't allowed to touch anything under the tree until everyone was awake and had gathered. It was a smart way to make sure they got a bit more of a lie-in. To assist in keeping us quiet, stockings had books, games, and food. There was the traditional orange along with a snack. I received PKU cookies I'd baked with mum the day before, or protein-free fruit jellies. As we grew older, my parents ensured the stocking included instructions on getting Christmas breakfast ready for them. Clever!

Thinking differently about Christmas

People often say that Christmas dinner is all about the turkey, which excludes vegetarians, vegans, and those on restricted diet therapies like PKU. But, I rarely come across people who actually have turkey. Every year, my friends discuss the various merits of lamb, goose, duck, pork, and beef wellington. There is always a conversation about the main PKU dish too.

As a child, I would regularly have my own stuffed vegetables. This meant I had something to carve at the Christmas table too. In more recent years, and with the availability of low protein pastry and cheese, I've tried new dishes. (*As product availability and ingredients do change, please take a look at my blog or other online sources for up-to-date ideas and recipes.*)

Suggestions for the main PKU dish:

- Vegetable wellington,
- Baked aubergine,
- BBQ Jackfruit, to emulate pulled pork.

Don't forget low-phe and protein-free trimmings like PKU-friendly Yorkshire puddings, sweet potato, parsnips, carrots, and sprouts. (*Recipes on www.pigpen.page*).

Christmas breakfast & snacks

Can you really go past pancakes or waffles as a Christmas breakfast treat? Plenty of PKU food companies offer recipes on making these with their products. Those on higher phe allowances may be able to buy gluten-free pancakes, waffles, or crumpets.

Food-less advent calendars, or calendars which you can purchase and then fill yourself, are a great help for those navigating Christmas with PKU (or any restricted diet). This is where online communities can help with sourcing little treats and gifts which are protein-free.

We all have our favourite Christmas Day snacks, and mine include avocado dips, semi-dried tomatoes, and plenty of exotic fruits like melon, pawpaw (papaya), and mango. We always buy phe-free fruit jellies to go with the chocolate covered ginger. These sweets last from Christmas Eve, to Boxing Day, and beyond.

If you are a baker, then the low protein food specialists have plenty of ideas for Christmas treats; including mince pies, and Christmas ginger biscuits. Again, I have not included recipes here, but see the links for updated websites. My main tip would be to ensure you have plenty of phe-free treats around to allow the traditional gorging with less of the guilt.

PKU adults and alcohol

Firstly, wine has no protein. I'll just say that again, wine has no protein. A can of beer is roughly 1 phe exchange, while a pint is starts from 1.5 phe. There is more protein in a Guinness or wheat beer, but these are rough guidelines.

Spirits or drinks which do not contain mixers with milk or cream, tend to have no protein. But you do have to be careful of any sodas or other mixers. Aspartame is always a lurking danger. Luckily, aspartame is the only artificial sweetener which we need to avoid. Saccharin, Acesulfame K, Sucralose, and Stevia are all permitted. Aspartame is being gradually phased out following some health fears. Several brands now offer aspartame-free sodas.

This is where a little time spent studying labels in a supermarket aisle for aspartame content may be helpful. Later, when ordering in a pub or club, try to get a quick glance over the bar. Fevertree tonic is aspartame-free, as are some Schweppes full fat varieties *(at time of publication)*.

Generally if the lemonade or coke is served from one of those ready-made taps then it is best avoided. Sorry, aspartame is everywhere. But, if the pub is quiet, bemused bartenders have been happy for me to have a brief look at the label on their mixer cans and bottles.

Tips for nights out with PKU

Everyone needs a celebration or a big night out, and those of us with PKU are no exception. The key is to make sensible choices early on. Simple things like having a phe-free meal or snack can help reduce your anxiety later. Making good decisions is easier on a full stomach.

Try to take your supplement early on. Once you have taken it, you can relax. If you forget, it isn't fun to take your supplement before collapsing into bed. But I promise you, after decades of trial and error, that you will feel much better in the morning for doing so.

If, like myself and many people, you will enjoy a glass and then switch to something alcohol-free, then there are still plenty of options. There are phe-free cordials which mix up well with sparkling water. I often have a lime and soda for a phe-and-alcohol-free celebratory drink.

This can be problematic in a bar, especially when the mixer comes out of the tap dispenser beloved by busy publicans. There is no way for someone with PKU to know if there is aspartame in there, and decades of questioning is yet to find a bar staff who knows the additive contents of the pre-mixed cordial. Furthermore, it is a rare bar person who takes kindly to interrogation over syrup ingredients at 11pm on a busy Friday night. This is where knowing the contents of your favourite mixer, or getting a taste for wine, can help.

27. Women and PKU

First, I will address the question: "why is there not a specific chapter for men?" It is both a legitimate query, and easily dealt with. There are two obvious and important concerns which women must manage, which do not directly affect men with PKU.

- Carrying a pregnancy.
- The monthly menstrual cycle.

A further argument could be made that other problems with managing PKU impact females to a greater degree than males. For example, a larger proportion of the work involved in managing a home & family, including food, tends to fall on women. Women tend to face stronger stigmas around body image and food behaviour, caused by years of societal pressure. While men suffer these pressures too, they continue to influence females more.

I note that I am unfamiliar with the male experience, and look forward to reading about PKU from a male perspective. This chapter will look at the two biological processes mentioned above.

Pregnancy

The essential message here, even if you read no further, is to get professional, clinical help if you have PKU and are considering a family. This support is essential from pre-conception though to breastfeeding. A healthy pregnancy is possible with PKU with planning and support. There is a list of support services at the end of this book.

Probability of child with PKU

In the general population, the probability of having a child with PKU is roughly 1 in 10,000. That does change with ethnicity, and there is ongoing research on this. However, that probability does increase when one of the parents has PKU themselves.

The genetics, a brief look

PKU is caused by an autosomal recessive genetic defect. There are complete definitions of that term available online, or in your high-school biology textbook. I will simply attempt to explain, in lay person's terms, what that means for PKU.

An autosome is a component of our genetic make up, part of our DNA. When these are copied from parent to child, there is a chance that there may be an error. Someone with PKU has inherited two slightly changed genetic autosomes, one from each parent. Everyone inherits these components. A person without PKU might have either two standard components, or one standard and one changed component. It is only when a person inherits two changed components that they have PKU.

The recessive part of the name comes from the fact that transfer of two changed components, and hence the incidence of PKU, is quite rare. That is, the standard components are far more likely to be passed on to any child.

However, a person with PKU doesn't have a standard component, so any child of someone with PKU is certain to inherit at least one changed component, and be a carrier. The chance of the child having PKU depends on which type of component is inherited from the other parent.

A parent without PKU may have two standard components, in which case the child will inherit one standard and one changed component, and will not have PKU. Or, the non-PKU parent may be a carrier, meaning they have one standard and one changed component. A carrier is more likely to pass on the standard component to any child, but it is possible that the changed component will be passed on.

Potential parents can be tested to determine whether they are carriers or not. There are several companies which offer this testing commercially. I have not been able to find any free carrier testing. The best source to find this type of testing would be your local PKU clinic, specialist, or support group.

Preconception to breast-feeding

It is important for someone with PKU who is planning for or expecting a child, to receive specialist clinic support. Ideally, this support would start before conception, but it is never too late to seek help. This support is to ensure that your baby is as healthy as possible, and that you, the mother, remain healthy during the pregnancy and breastfeeding.

The advice and research on pregnancy and PKU is constantly updated and revised. This is why the advice in this book is to seek help for the latest information and support. Please contact your current PKU clinic for help, or use the *Resources* at the end of the book to find a new one. Pregnancy is a critical time for the health of a baby, and for parents. Please reach out for specialist support.

Periods and PKU

Some may not think that managing PKU during periods requires any attention. But then, the menstrual cycle has been stigmatised and ignored for far too long.

On average, periods start between 11 & 14 years of age, and continue until the early 50s (Holland, 2018). This means women are likely to have 450 periods across their lifetime. There are aspects of menstrual cycles which are consistent from person to person, but there are also differences. Cycle length is one of these variables.

My university flat was all female, and one night we had the inevitable conversation about synching. This is the phenomenon whereby menstruating females who live together might find that their menstrual cycles synchronise, and they ovulate and menstruate at the same time. There were six of us in the flat, and our cycles represented a neat, if tiny, bell curve. Four had the standard 28-day cycle, or bled one week in every four. One bled every 5 weeks, and one every three.

Far from simply being an interesting anecdote, this had real implications. One flatmate would spend roughly 18 weeks of the year on her period, with all the associated pain, discomfort, and hormonal changes. Another would only bleed for 10 weeks of the year. This variation meant the flatmates had markedly different experiences in everything from health, through productivity, to lifestyle.

However, this is merely an anecdote. We require scientific data to remain objective when looking at the effect of PKU on the menstrual cycle. Sadly, there isn't any. Or rather, there is very little.

Published research on PKU and periods

I found only one reference which might help someone to manage their PKU across the menstrual cycle. One line in a single paper which mentions something which half of us with PKU will need to manage for decades. A UK clinician pointed me towards another reference, but I simply could not find it.

A few papers mentioned, in passing, that some with PKU have menstrual irregularities. These included the absence of periods, or irregular cycles. Most researchers attributed this to high phe levels and moved on. While the menstrual cycle was mentioned in a significant number of papers, the research focused on pregnancy with PKU. And for good reason, it is an area in need of important and critical research.

Why was there so little focus on managing the menstrual cycle with PKU? This is a neglected question, with possible answers in gender bias which go beyond the scope of this book. Indeed, there is an award-winning book on gender bias in research; Invisible Women by Caroline Criado Perez.

Teasing out what we can

Let's look at what we do have. The reference I found noted that there might be fluctuations in blood phe levels during the menstrual cycle, and that higher blood phe levels are likely in the late-luteal phase. (MacLeod & Ney, 2010) There are a few key phrases which we need to look at here.

The luteal phase of the menstrual cycle usually lasts two weeks, and is the time between ovulation and the first day of your period. Therefore the late luteal phase is the week before your period starts.

The one bit of scientific advice I could find on managing PKU and your period warns us that blood phe levels are likely to rise in the week before your period. Right when the hormones kick in and start to affect your mood, body temperature, and appetite.

This isn't intended to make you gloomy. I hope to highlight something which may be useful, something which I wish I had known years ago. Because when you know about something, you can plan for it. I have lived with PKU and a menstrual cycle for nearly three decades now. These are a few suggestions based on this experience.

- Track your menstrual cycle. Even 30 years on, it can still be a surprise when the period turns up. This is a way to turn hindsight (wishing you had phe-free snacks ready), into foresight (buying phe-free snacks in advance.) Simple changes like this can make a marked difference to phe levels on a daily and weekly basis. New apps help with period tracking, and many can act as both a guide and a reminder.

- Work out your symptoms, and find phe-free remedies. While menstrual cycles can directly affect our appetites, there are other ways in which the cycle may ultimately impact blood phe levels. Even women without PKU report difficulties in regulating body temperature in the late luteal phase. They have trouble staying warm, and are driven to hot food and drinks in the days before a period. These provide other ways in which high blood phe levels might creep in; it is difficult to make a good decision on phe intake while cold and in pain. These decisions are easier with a plan in place. You might wear warmer clothing, have phe-free food and drink available, exercise inside instead of in the cold.

This chapter is shorter, far shorter, than it should be. However, as I detailed above, anything further would be anecdotal, rather than scientific. It is to be hoped that new research will be available for any future edition of this book.

28. Healthy eating and exercise with PKU

How to eat healthily with PKU; how to exercise safely with PKU; how to lose weight with PKU… I can't recall a single PKU gathering, webinar, cooking event, or conference which didn't address at least one of these issues.

This might seem odd. The limitations of a restricted diet therapy mean our diet is fundamentally based on fruit and vegetables. This appears healthy to strangers and passing acquaintances. An order of a salad is often followed by the comment, "that sounds like a healthy diet."

The critical thing to remember is that exercise is as important for someone with PKU as it is for anyone else, and it is just as safe. Likewise, healthy eating and safe weight loss are definitely possible while following the restricted diet therapy.

Why, then, are these questions of healthy eating, weight loss, and exercise so prevalent in the PKU community? If you are struggling with any of these issues while on a restricted diet therapy, then you are not alone. Research published in 2013 shows that those in the UK with PKU have the same levels of obesity and elevated weights as the general population (Robertson et al., 2013).

This shows that the questions of healthy eating, exercise, and weight loss are not unique to the PKU population. These are issues with which society at large is grappling. Crucially, the restricted diet treatment magnifies these difficulties for us.

Healthy eating with PKU

The challenge of healthy eating is harder when on the restricted diet therapy. If we are already limited to only 15% of foods, there is less variety to work with. This means it is crucial to look at what we are eating, and when. Managing PKU means we must count the amount of phe we eat. Because of our restrictions, it may be easy to over eat, or gorge on, low-phe & phe-free foods.

However, there are still calories in phe-free and low-phe foods. That might seem obvious, but it is worth remembering. The restricted diet therapy means that someone with PKU might place a high value on phe-free foods, and forget about the other nutrients and fats they contain.

Take this example, which is straight out of my playbook. I will often tackle the afternoon munchies with phe-free biscuits. These might be homemade or supplied by one of the specialised food manufacturers. In my head they are a safe option, and I have finished a whole box or batch in one sitting. But, while I might be avoiding phe, I will still be eating large amounts of calories.

The trick is to use our phe allowance for healthy options which fill us up. Now, a dark chocolate digestive is a treat, but contains about one phe. Plus, it is hard to stop at one digestive! Even if you manage to do so, a single biscuit is hardly filling. The lowest protein coconut yoghurt I have managed to find is 160g for one phe. This is far more filling, and the basis for a PKU-friendly meal. Add in some fresh fruit and that is breakfast. Or swirl in honey for a dessert.

Some other suggestions might be snacking on popcorn, using one phe worth of cream cheese as a dip for carrot or celery sticks, or using pine nuts to add phe and crunch to a salad or pasta dish.. You don't have to avoid biscuits all the time, perhaps save them for a weekend treat?

One of the reasons someone on the restricted diet therapy might eat more than the standard portion is that reaching satiety can be difficult. I've offered a few tips on finding satiety in *PKU and being Hangry*.

Weight loss and PKU

"Once you've filled in the form, we'll get your weight, height, & BMI." Ah, the loaded question: what is my BMI today? Like many with PKU, every clinic visit means another round of body measurements. I don't weigh myself in between, but, I have been unable to avoid the scales and height measures.

As a result of decades in PKU clinics, I have an extensive record of my BMI going back many years. While I try not to obsess about weight, I have never escaped the scales. This routine of measurements leads, inevitably, to some form of judgement. This may never be said aloud, the judgement may just be the voice in my head automatically noting an increase. But, it is a judgement nonetheless.

At my first PKU clinic after joining a gym, I was quietly confident. It had been six months since my last encounter with the scales, and I had been fairly active in that time. My clothes were looser, and I was completing my regular exercise class without resorting to the easy options. I felt slimmer, fitter, and stronger. I was sure I weighed less; the question was: how much had I lost?

Nothing. The scales said my weight and BMI had actually gone up slightly. Three hundred grams gained, confidence lost. How did that happen! I was fitter and stronger. It is an old saying that muscle weighs more than fat; was that the explanation? Perhaps I was simply reading too much into one measurement.

Beyond BMI

We need to consider other measures, not just BMI, when assessing our physical health. The NHS advises that, while BMI lets you know if you weigh too much, it can't tell if you have an excess of fat. Put simply, this calculation of weight and height does not distinguish between the proportions of fat, muscle, or bone in the body.

Essentially, BMI measures if you are carrying too much weight for your height. It can't tell you if that weight is excess fat or excess muscle. This is why athletes and gym bunnies are sometimes categorised as obese under the BMI system. It is their muscle which has caused them to be that heavy. This is an important point; BMI just indicates healthy weight across a population. BMI is not a personalised reminder of your chocolate and/or beer binges. It lets you know roughly how you are doing.

Another measurement which can help is the circumference of the waist. Again, it only gives an indication, but a significant one. If you carry too much fat around your stomach, this increases your health risk. As a rough guide, the circumference of your waist should be less than half of your height. E.g., someone who is 160 cm tall would ideally have a waist circumference of less than 80 cm.

Safe weight loss and PKU diets

Losing weight quickly is not a great plan. The term 'yoyo dieting' is commonly used to describe those times when we work hard to lose weight only to see it all come back on again later. Slow and steady changes in habit and lifestyle are best. There is a consensus among registered dieticians and personal trainers that we should be aiming for a safe rate of weight loss of between 0.5 kg and 1 kg per week. That's between around 1lb and 2lb a week (NHS website 2, n.d.)

We can work to that guideline, but bear in mind that those of us with PKU are already on a restrictive diet. Watching what we eat and counting intake is a daily necessity and we already eat a rigid diet with little room to manoeuvre. Not many on PKU treatment will have the quick weight-loss option of removing visits to the kebab shop.

We also need to remember that, just as putting weight on can be a slow process, losing weight will take time. My handy spreadsheet tells me that the last time I was close to the healthy BMI range, Kate Winslet and Leonardo Di Caprio were running about on the set of Titanic. This slow accretion of weight gain will not be countered overnight. That is an important point to remember as we grapple with all the judgement and shame associated with weight and food.

We need to make changes which we can maintain over the long term, and accept that this is about a change over months, rather than reaching 'ideal weight' in a matter of weeks. With little to cut out of an already restricted diet, that means making healthier food choices, and getting more active.

PKU and exercise

Exercise is as essential for someone with PKU as it is for anyone. Unfortunately, those of us with PKU face the same problem with motivation as others. Occasionally, it is just too easy not to exercise. I am one of those who will always find a reason why now is not the best time to go for a run or do body strength exercises: "I'm on my period." "I am too busy". "The weather is too hot / too cold / too wet…"

Here is the secret. There is no magic button to make you fitter. There is no perfect moment you should wait for. When it comes to fitness, sometimes you just have to do it. Often you will feel better afterwards. This is a known, if odd, phenomenon where the motivation comes after the exercise. That knowledge may not help you off the sofa on day one. But the memory of how you felt after exercise, and the sense of achievement, will help with day two.

Fuelling exercise on the PKU diet

Like many people, I took up running when the gyms closed during the pandemic. After a month or two of these runs, I was getting a few niggles and pains. As is so often the case, anxiety kicked in and my first thought was that I had screwed up on the restricted diet therapy. A quick email with the dieticians confirmed that the supplement I was on didn't need adjusting.

The important message from the clinic was that taking the supplements immediately after exercise has more benefit than taking them before. And when exercise last for less than an hour, we shouldn't need to add any more meals and snacks to our diets.

This is true even for muscle building. I started doing yoga as part of my recovery from an unrelated injury. Years of cycling and football meant that I resembled a T. rex. Good leg strength, puny arm muscles.

The planking, push-ups, and balancing exercises involved in Vinyasa flow yoga have greatly improved my upper-body strength. You don't need to be taking protein-packed power drinks to build muscle. Our supplement is already a power drink! It is a relief to note that a few tweaks to when we eat and take supplements is enough to support the type of strength & muscle building which most people require.

The key is to refuel with the right food at the right time

Many gym or fitness apps & programmes include a food plan. While these are generally unsuitable for those of us with PKU, we do need to think about the food we eat after working out.

It is important to fuel our bodies after exercise, to stave off hunger and to help the muscles to repair and strengthen.

A crucial component of this refuelling with PKU is the supplements. These supplements have already been prescribed for you to support a healthy lifestyle. Think of them as your ready-made nutrient pack, your go-to fuel after hitting the gym or any form of exercise.

Ideally, we will take our supplement and have a meal, with a portion of our phe allowance, within one hour after exercise. Everyone I've spoken to, from clinicians to personal trainers with PKU, agreed that this is the optimal way to refuel after exercise.

If the supplement you are currently on is not suitable for you to take within an hour after exercise, you may want to try another. There are many formats and flavours of supplement available, and there is more information in the chapters on supplements.

Cardio vs Strength

A favourite topic in many discussions on exercise is whether cardio is better than strengthening exercises. In fact, you need both forms of exercise in a healthy lifestyle. This is true for people with PKU too.

To recap, cardio exercises may be described as catabolic, where your body is breaking down tissue (hopefully fat!). This process is called catabolism and may cause blood phe levels to increase following intensive periods of cardio exercise.

However, this would require intense cardio exercise over a long time. This means far more cardio than someone might do to meet daily exercise guidelines.

Strength exercises like push-ups or weightlifting have an anabolic effect. These may reduce blood phe levels because the body is taking phe out of the blood to build new muscle.

There is a little more on the effects which the anabolic and catabolic processes can have in *What else affects blood phe levels?*.

However, someone who is on the correct phe allowance and supplement intake should not have a problem with blood phe changes when undertaking a regular amount of daily exercise.

Part six: Beyond restricted diet therapy

29. Other treatments in use globally

I wrote at the start that there was nothing our parents or grandparents did which led to our PKU. That all we can do is make the best of it, and press for better treatments.

The 21st century has seen the development and use of treatments for PKU which move beyond the restricted diet therapy. Despite the long wait, many patients still need to advocate for access to these new treatments. However, there is progress.

Large Neutral Amino Acid (LNAA) treatment

This is a supplementary therapy for PKU used in some European countries and is particularly aimed at those with mild PKU. The mechanism in LNAA treatment relies on the competition between molecules for passage from the blood into the brain. This passage is protected by the blood/brain barrier, which acts like a security system.

Remember, it is high phe in the brain which causes problems. We measure phe levels in the blood, because we can't yet measure the amount of phe directly in the brain.

Phe is one of nine LNAAs which pass across the blood/brain barrier. In people with PKU, high levels of phe in the blood mean that a higher percentage of the LNAAs crossing into the brain are phe. The idea of LNAA treatment is to change the percentage of phe molecules passing into the brain by increasing the levels of other LNAAs in the blood. This would return the ratio of LNAAs in the blood closer to equilibrium, which removes the advantage which phe molecules have at the blood/brain barrier. A study published in 2020 found that adding in LNAA supplements along with a restricted diet therapy tended to improve both adherence to treatment and the quality of life for those who participated (Burlina, et al., 2020).

LNAA could, in theory, be administered alongside the restricted diet therapy or other treatments for PKU. However, the difficulty lies in proving the effect. For decades, we have measured the severity of someone's PKU and the possible effect on their brain through blood phe levels.

In LNAA treatment, the idea is to remove this relationship so that blood phe levels no longer provide a window on the amount of phe reaching the brain. This removes the main objective scientific measurement relied on over decades of PKU treatment. So, how do we prove that LNAA treatment is safe through objective measures?

I have had no experience with LNAA treatment, but it is considered an option for adults in European countries such as Denmark. I suspect that a key hurdle in government commissioning elsewhere will be the need to find a clinical measurement of the treatment benefit, as blood phe measurements may not be considered an effective measure for this LNAA treatment.

To sapropterin, and beyond

In December 2021, the body which governs clinical commissioning in the UK approved the use of sapropterin, commonly known as Kuvan. This marked the first time that a treatment beyond the restricted diet therapy was approved for PKU in the UK. Brits with PKU had spent 68 years managing a treatment which was first developed in the year that Queen Elizabeth II was crowned.

This development did not come easily. There were 12 years of lobbying to fund this new treatment. The celebration is long overdue, but must be cautious. Sapropterin will have an undeniable influence on the lives of those for whom it works. However, due to the nature of its action, the drug may only work for 1 in 4 of those with PKU. I explain why below. First, why all the different names for this treatment?

Sapropterin aka Kuvan aka BH4 aka...

Which name is correct? These names are being used interchangeably, though they do refer to different things. It comes down to the difference between the name of the medicine, and brand names. Much like Panadol is one common brand name for the painkiller paracetamol. The terms are often used interchangeably, but have separate meanings. It can be confusing, so here is a quick guide.

Kuvan is a brand name which the company BioMarin uses for sapropterin. Other companies may produce branded forms of sapropterin, so there may be other brand names for this medicine soon.

Note: BioMarin is not the company which has the contract with the NHS in England at the time of writing. The drug initially made available on the NHS will come from the company called Teva. It will be a generic, non-branded form of sapropterin. Those prescribed sapropterin in England will not see 'Kuvan' on the label, just as the own-brand paracetamol in supermarkets does not call itself 'Panadol'.

Sapropterin is the medicine, and the full name is sapropterin dihydrochloride. Just as paracetamol is the medicine in Panadol, sapropterin is the medicine in Kuvan. Sapropterin comes as a pill to be swallowed at the time and dosage prescribed by a PKU specialist. The dosage is worked out based on bodyweight and other factors.

Where does BH4 come from? Sapropterin is a synthetic version of an enzyme co-factor (and I will explain what that is soon). The enzyme co-factor of interest here is called '6R-tetrahydrobiopterin', or '6R-BH4'. It is from this that we get the shortened term BH4.

Clear as mud, right? From now on, this book will use the term sapropterin, so as not to confuse anyone using generic pills or different brand names. The paragraph above included the term enzyme co-factor, and to explain what that is, we need to go into how sapropterin works.

How does sapropterin work?

Sapropterin is an enzyme co-factor. An enzyme co-factor is a non-protein chemical that assists the enzyme with its biological reaction. In this instance, 6R-BH4 is a substance which helps the enzyme PAH to break down phe.

This is why those researching new PKU treatments were interested. The researchers found that they could create a synthetic version of this 6R-BH4 chemical in a form which was suitable for a medicine. They created the medicine known as sapropterin.

In simple terms, sapropterin boosts the efficiency of any existing PAH. This is one reason why it has varying effects in different patients. If someone only has a small amount of PAH, there is not much for the sapropterin to boost. This is why the treatment tends to work best in those with mild or moderate PKU.

The NSPKU estimate that 20-30% of patients with mild or moderate PKU may respond to sapropterin (NSPKU, 2017). However, because of the wide variance in PKU mutations, there is a chance that someone with more severe PKU may respond to sapropterin.

Will sapropterin work for me?

It is possible to use genetic phenotype testing to establish which patients may respond. Most clinicians will also use a challenge trial as well, where the person with PKU is trailed on sapropterin for a time and carefully monitored for any effects. The cost of this genetic phenotype testing, and the length and conditions of any trial period, vary across countries and health regimes. For that reason, please do contact your clinic or local patient organisation; I have provided some links in *Resources*.

The good news is that sapropterin is not the only new development in PKU treatment.

PEG-PAL, an injection for PKU

Those with PKU and their families are constantly on the lookout for new ways to manage PKU. We may come across stories of an injection which means someone with PKU can eat a more normal diet.

This may sound like a magical fantasy, but there is an injection for PKU. Only, it isn't magic and does have side effects of significant concern. This injection is known variously as Palynziq, or PegPal, and is more common in the USA. As I prepared this book for publication, news broke that PEG-PAL is unlikely to be available on the UK health system in the foreseeable future.

PAL aka PEG-PAL aka Pegvaliase aka Palynziq...

Yes, here is another new treatment for PKU which has a confusing series of names. As with sapropterin, these four names refer to different aspects of a single method of treatment. Unlike sapropterin, this is not an enzyme cofactor which is taken in pill form. This is an enzyme replacement therapy which is usually injected.

What do all these names mean?

PAL is the enzyme. PAL stands for phenylalanine ammonia-lyase, which is a common enzyme in many plant species. As a quick reminder, there are many enzymes which each breakdown different amino acids in protein. People with PKU cannot produce enough of the enzyme phenylalanine hydroxylase, or PAH.

The similarity in these two enzyme names is no coincidence, both of them break down phenylalanine (phe). PAL does in plants what PAH does in humans. But PAL breaks the amino acid down differently. Fortunately, the different reaction results in end products which are easily processed in humans. This is why it has been developed as a treatment for PKU.

PEG-PAL, or the stealth enzyme. The addition of PEG in front of PAL in this term indicates that the enzyme PAL has been mixed with polyethylene glycol (PEG). PEG is a compound which is safe for humans to consume and is commonly used in medicine.

In this case, the PEG is used to disguise the PAL enzyme from the immune system. Remember that PAL is an enzyme found in plants, so it is foreign to the human body. If it were injected without PEG, then the immune system would see the enzyme as a threat and destroy it. PEG-PAL is basically the enzyme in stealth mode, able to hide from the immune system and get to work. However, the stealth coating doesn't always work, and this can lead to side effects.

Pegvaliase and Palynziq are brand names. BioMarin have developed PEG-PAL into an injectable treatment for PKU. Initially, this was called 'Pegvaliase' but it is now called

'Palynziq'. Essentially, Pegvaliase and Palynziq are brand names for the treatment PEG-PAL; in the same way that Panadol is a brand name for paracetamol.

It is worth noting that BioMarin are the same company which make Kuvan, the branded form of sapropterin which remained too expensive for the UK health system. Eventually, generic sapropterin pills were developed, which were much cheaper. It is to be hoped that generic forms of PEG-PAL may also become available at some point. To avoid more confusion, this book will use the term PEG-PAL.

Does PEG-PAL work?

To recap the above, PAL is an enzyme which algae use to process phe. PEG-PAL is that enzyme in a form which can be injected into the human body. Once there, it can remove the phe which is not processed in someone with PKU. There is some evidence which shows that PKU patients, who were not maintaining the European blood phe targets, were able to reach those levels using PEG-PAL. Excitingly, the treatment also allowed some eat a nearly normal diet. That is encouraging; however:

Problems with using PEG-PAL

PAL is a plant enzyme and is not recognised by the human body. Even with the stealth coating offered by PEG, this origin causes problems during treatment. The human immune system views PEG-PAL as a foreign chemical, so treatment produces side effects. BioMarin's own website notes some of these common side effects as:

- anaphylaxis and/or skin allergy reactions
- joint and head pains;
- nausea, stomach pain, and vomiting. (BioMarin, n.d.)

This is not the full list. The worst risk is that of anaphylaxis, or severe allergic reaction, which may be life-threatening.

Participants in the study mentioned above had an unusually high number of side effects. A third of the study participants had such bad reactions that they dropped out of the trial despite the increased diet freedom. That means the reactions certainly weren't just a small irritation. It would take a lot for someone who had been able to eat most foods to go back to a heavily restricted diet.

What next? More Science!

In May 2019, the European Commission granted BioMarin permission to market Palynziq in the EU for the limited treatment of some PKU patients who meet certain criteria. Basically, they were allowed to open treatment to patients with PKU over 16 years old who had blood phe levels greater than 600μmol/L, despite being on diet.

But there are no studies into the effect that this enzyme will have over a longer time. It is possible that the immune system could fight back so much that the injected enzyme becomes ineffective. Is it worth all that pain only to end up back where you started? There are some big unknowns here and, as ever with science, more studies are needed.

30. Living with PKU in the future

After nearly 70 years of working on the restricted diet therapy, research has moved to alternative treatments for PKU. Some of those now available have been outlined in Other treatments in use globally. Here are some possibilities which are under development at the time of writing. This list is hopeful, but all treatments are in their early stages. It is not known if they will work, or what the longterm effects might be.

Gut absorption therapy in PKU

There are a few options under investigation which might absorb phe from food in the digestive system. This would prevent the excess phe from transferring into the bloodstream, and then the brain. One option is using a safe version of E. coli to carry PAH, the enzyme which people with PKU are lacking, into the digestive tract.

In July 2021, one synthetic biology company revealed that their treatment along these lines did not cause immediate problems in a 4-day trial (Gen website, 2021). It wasn't noted whether the therapy had any effect on blood levels of phe, just that there were no immediate harmful effects in that short trial. There is a long way from here to a new therapy for PKU available to patients, but it is an encouraging step.

Another option might be to use a medical resin, instead of bacteria, to deliver the enzyme into the gut. It is very early days for both methods, and we just don't know if either approach is safe or if it will be effective.

Other enzyme replacement therapies

This branch of research looks at using a substitute enzyme to help someone with PKU to metabolise phe. PEG-PAL uses this form of treatment, introducing an enzyme to the body which can then break down the excess phe. There is now research into the possibility of introducing engineered cells to the liver. These cells would then deliver the replacement enzyme directly to the digestive system. Again, this is very new. One of the key questions is working out how long such manipulated liver cells might live, and thus how effective any treatment might be.

Gene therapy

In early 2020, the news there may be a gene therapy trial in the UK caused quite a stir at the NSPKU conference. The Covid-19 pandemic then struck, and I have not heard news on this approach since. However, in lay person terms, this therapy would involve:

- Isolating the bit of the gene which corrects the production of PAH.
- Finding a (good!) virus to carry the gene safely and without alteration.
- Finding a way to inject the virus carrier and gene into someone with PKU.
- Directing the virus carrier to the correct place in the body for it to work.
- Once in place, triggering the gene segment into action.

Only after all these steps have happened safely and effectively would the gene segments produce PAH and treat the PKU. Ensuring the steps can happen safely and reliably many times over is no easy task. The researchers do know that the immune system will react to the virus. It is the job of the immune system to react to every virus.

This mixture may be injected into someone and fail. Or it may work for a year or two before stopping, and the reaction of the immune system may mean that it is not possible to try again.

While the hope is for a lifelong cure, we currently have no idea if that will actually happen. I don't pretend to know all the variables, but reproducibility and safety are troubling unknowns at this point. This is, to varying degrees, true for all treatments for PKU.

Reproducibility & safety

The hope that these potential treatments inspire in someone with PKU is difficult to express. This is a hope shared by all affected families, and by their clinicians too. Every health care worker I have ever met wants to do their best for the patient.

That may not always be obvious to the patient, and it must be difficult to be the objective person in the room. The person to say 'wait, please!' when others are reaching for a new treatment which may be life-changing or dangerous, or both.

The promise in all the potential therapies mentioned above, and others which may be underway, is exciting. But, as always in science, there are many 'buts'. There are still many unknowns about these technologies, such as:

- Will the therapy work? Not just in a few people in laboratory conditions, but over time in a wide and varying population who are living imperfect lives in an imperfect world?
- What is the correct dose for each therapy? Does the dose requirement differ between patients, or between different

life stages e.g., between a child and an adult, and what about pregnant woman?
- Does the effectiveness of the dose diminish over time, meaning the patient needs exponentially more treatment for the same results? Can any required dose be administered in a safe and consistent way?
- What are the side effects of the therapy? Every medicine has some side effects, are those produced by this treatment manageable? What about rare but critical side effects which may not show up in small trials, but cause problems when a higher number of people are treated? Does treatment adversely affect other organs, or interfere with treatments for other conditions?

These are only the questions which I have. Experienced researchers will have many more questions to answer, then there will be the difficulties thrown up in the progress of research. There is an enormous amount of work going into all of these areas, and it all comes back to the need for...

More research

Research into all of these potential new therapies, and others, are ongoing. If you would like to stay in touch with developments, one of the best ways I've found to do so is to join an organisation which campaigns for new PKU treatments. This means that you are in contact with others who are following the same developments, and may hear if there are trials planned in your area.

Bear in mind that not everyone with PKU will be eligible for trials. This has happened to me several times. Sadly, someone who has worked to maintain blood phe levels within the European guidelines for years was not eligible for the early sapropterin or PEG-PAL trials.

This could be interpreted as requiring people with PKU to risk brain damage to be considered for one of the non-diet therapy trials. That feels incredibly unfair, even before one delves into the ethical issues! Sticking to the restricted diet therapy is terribly difficult, whatever your blood phe levels are. To work so hard, and then be excluded from possible new therapies for doing well, is extremely disappointing. I would like to see all varieties of PKU and PKU management to be included in research in future.

We all deserve access to better PKU foods, medicines, and treatments. But we need to be aware that sapropterin, PEG-PAL and other new PKU treatments may not work for everyone. Further, the long-term consequences of these therapies are unknown.

PKU is caused by a mutation, of which there are hundreds of different variations. Short of a complete, life-long correction at the genetic level, no single treatment will work for everyone. The variety of people living with PKU means we need a multitude of therapies, a buffet of treatments. From this, we might work with our clinicians to select therapies which complement each other, and make it easier to live with PKU.

It is with that hope in mind that this book ends with the cry of scientists across the years: More research is required!

Thank you for reading.

You can sign up for more on PKU, including recipes & research updates at: www.pigpen.page/newsletter

Part seven: Resources

Units used

g gram: e.g., 10g is 10 grams

mg milligrams: e.g., 10 mg is 10 milligrams

µmol/L micro moles per litre: e.g., 250 µmol/L means there are 250 µmoles of phe in every litre of blood. In some countries, including the US, blood phe levels are reported in mg/dL. As an example: the range 120-360 µmol/L may also be expressed as 1.35-4 mg/dL. This book will use the measurement of µmol/L.

Resources

Abbreviations & Acronyms

For an explanation of these terms, please see Glossary

CBT Cognitive Behavioural Therapy

GMP Glycomacropeptide

HPA Hyperphenylalaninemia

IEM Inborn Error of Metabolism

IMD Inherited Metabolic Disorder

LNAAs Large Neutral Amino Acids

low-phe A food or drink considered free of phenylalanine

PAH Phenylalanine hydroxylase

phe Phenylalanine

phe-free A food or drink considered free of Phenylalanine

PKU Phenylketonuria

Tyr Tyrosine

PKU Support and Patient groups

UK

NSPKU: The National Society for Phenylketonuria. https://www.nspku.org/

A UK-based organisation formed to support people with PKU, and actively promote new research and treatments. The

NSPKU also advocate on behalf of those with PKU. They have lobbied MPs, and reported to NHS committees to campaign for PKU treatments beyond the restricted diet therapy in the UK.

The society have a website & monthly magazine. A crucial part aim is to support families with new diagnosis, and assisting people with PKU to manage the restricted diet therapy. They raise money to pay for phe analysis. The society also provide resources such as lists of low-phe and phe-free supermarket foods, and provide assistance for clinicians and GPs who may be learning about PKU alongside their patient.

The NSPKU have a helpline for UK numbers: 030 3040 1090. Or see more ways to contact them here: https://www.nspku.org/contact-us/. Calls to the above numbers will probably be charged, but they have a call back service on their website. They also have a page specifically for those with a newly diagnosed baby: https://www.nspku.org/new-diagnosis-of-pku-2/

MSUK: Metabolic Support UK. https://www.metabolicsupportuk.org/

Metabolic Support UK is a patient organisation for Inherited Metabolic Disorders. The organisation has developed over the years to become part of a worldwide collaborative network of groups and organisations, ensuring it is at the forefront of developments such as newborn screening and treatments.

EU

PKU Association of Ireland. http://pku.ie/

The PKU Association of Ireland was set up to help & support those affected by PKU, and other metabolic disorders that can be managed in the same way as PKU (E.g., HPA0). They

Resources

share stories, advice, tips, and recipes and a supportive environment for help with PKU.

ESPKU: The European Society for PKU and allied disorders treated as PKU. https://www.espku.org/

That is one of the longest names for an organisation which I have come across, but it suits an umbrella organisation. The ESPKU is a grouping of national and regional associations which were created by parents across 31 countries. The reference to 'allied disorders' in the name means they represent a number of other Inherited Metabolic Disorders alongside PKU.

The member organisations directory is a superb resource for both national PKU organisations and specialist food companies in the EU. Find your national or regional organisation here: https://www.espku.org/who-we-are/interesting-stuff/

USA

NPKUA: National PKU Alliance. https://www.npkua.org/

The NPKUA is a national patient charity in the US which works for PKU research and advocates at a national level. Their resources page provides information on clinics, insurance coverage, finding foods, and financial aid. https://www.npkua.org/Resources

National PKU News. https://pkunews.org/

A website dedicated to providing resources and support for those with PKU and other IMD's. They launched the 'HowMuchPhe.org' service to make low-phe food lists available widely available. https://howmuchphe.org/

PKU and Me. https://www.pku.com/

This is a website sponsored by BioMarin as part of their RareConnections initiative. The aim is to provide guidance and support for healthy living with PKU.

Canada

CanPKU. https://canpku.org/

Based in Toronto, the Canadian PKU and Allied Disorders Inc. is a volunteer-led organisation with the aim of improving the lives of people with PKU. Their PKU resources page has numerous downloads in English and French to help families with PKU. https://www.canpku.org/Downloadable-educational-resources

Australia & Aotearoa/NZ

PKUNSW. https://www.pkunsw.org.au/

PKU Association of New South Wales has members is all Australian states and provides resources, news, and events for Aussie families with PKU.

Australasian Society for Inborn Errors of Metabolism (ASIEM). https://www.hgsa.org.au/asiem

A special interest group of scientists and health professionals who are involved in treating IMD's. They have produced a PKU Handbook and food resources which are available at: https://www.hgsa.org.au/resources/asiem-resources-for-parents-and-families/asiem-dietary-handbooks-and-protein-counting-resources

Global Online Community

I would suggest using the list above to find a patient organisation in your area and start by following their channel on your social media platform.

Resources

Possible financial support

Available support can change with each administration, I strongly urge you to contact a patient or charity support group for accurate information.

USA

'Help with bills' advice: https://www.usa.gov/help-with-bills

UK

Personal Independence Payment (PIP): https://www.gov.uk/pip

Ireland

Long-Term Illness Scheme: https://www.citizensinformation.ie/en/health/drugs_and_medicines/long_term_illness_scheme.html

Australia

Inborn Errors of Metabolism program: https://www.health.gov.au/initiatives-and-programs/inborn-errors-of-metabolism-program?utm_source=health.gov.au&utm_medium=callout-auto-custom&utm_campaign=digital_transformation

Aotearoa/NZ

WINZ Disability allowance: https://www.workandincome.govt.nz/products/a-z-benefits/disability-allowance.html

Support for returning to treatment

UK

In the UK, the NSPKU have information on returning to diet at https://www.nspku.org/wp-content/uploads/2020/02/Returning_to_PKU_diet.pdf

Or you can contact them for confidential support: They have a helpline for UK numbers: 030 3040 1090, or see more ways to contact them here: https://www.nspku.org/contact-us/. Calls to the above numbers will probably be charged, but they have a call back service on their website.

Ireland

The PKU Association of Ireland includes helpful links on their Resources page: http://pku.ie/resources/.

Or Nutricia Ireland offer return to diet information on their website at https://www.nutricia.ie/patients-carers/articles-stories/returning-to-diet.html.

The National Centre for Inherited Metabolic Disorders (NCIMD) in Ireland is located at Children's University Hospital, Temple Street, Dublin. The centre is also known as the Metabolic Unit. They have online and downloadable resources for PKU patients and family at https://metabolic.ie/patient-family-information/metabolic-conditions/phenylketonuria/

US

National PKU Alliance run both a 'Return to treatment' programme, and a 'Back to Care' programme: https://

Resources

www.npkua.org/Resources/Return-to-Treatment and http://adultswithpku.org/Back-to-Care

Specialist food companies with information

Nutricia UK: https://www.nutricia.co.uk/patients-carers/articles-stories/returning-to-diet.html#

Cambrooke UK: https://cambrooketherapeutics.co.uk/a-pku-return-and-the-benefits-paul-mckellar/

Find a clinic

UK

You can get a referral to an NHS PKU clinic through your local GP, and the NSPKU can help with this. The NSPKU have a helpline for UK numbers: 030 3040 1090. Calls may be charged, but they have a call back service and other ways to contact them at: https://www.nspku.org/contact-us/

US

National PKU Alliance, find a clinic page: https://www.npkua.org/Resources/Find-a-Clinic

Support for pregnancy

There is little information online dedicated to maternal PKU as pregnancy deserves specialised support. The best source of for help with a PKU pregnancy is your local specialist or clinic.

Information on genetics and inheritance patterns

Genetic Alliance UK website: Inheritance patterns page: https://geneticalliance.org.uk/information/learn-about-genetics/inheritance-patterns/

UK support

NSPKU Maternal PKU help: https://www.nspku.org/maternal-pku/

NSPKU Emergency Contacts: https://www.nspku.org/emergency-contacts/

USA

NPKUA website at https://www.npkua.org/What-is-PKU/About-PKU

Resources

Phe-free food lists

UK

NSPKU website, the documents page: https://www.nspku.org/documents/?wpdmc=dietary-info

Ireland

The National Centre for Inherited Metabolic Disorders (NCIMD) website: https://metabolic.ie/patient-family-information/metabolic-conditions/phenylketonuria/

EU

The best way to find food lists for EU countries is to find the national organisation. Fortunately, there is a handy list of member organisations on the ESPKU website:

https://www.espku.org/who-we-are/interesting-stuff/

US

The NPKUA website has a resource page with video supermarket guides and links to cookbooks & shopping guides. https://www.npkua.org/Resources

The 'How much phe' website is a subscription service which provides access to phe content in foods. https://howmuchphe.org/

Resources

Canada

The CanPKU website has downloadable patient resources which include food logs and help sheets. There are also guides to help families and friends to support someone with PKU at different life stages. https://canpku.org/Education-Patient-Support

Australia and Aotearoa/NZ

PKU Association of NSW: https://www.pkunsw.org.au/pku-friendly-products

Treatment manufacturers

Global websites

Biomarin: https://www.biomarin.com/our-motivation/diseases-and-conditions/pku/

Metax: https://www.metax.org/

Mevalia: https://www.mevalia.com/

Nutricia: https://www.nutricia.com/world.html

Prekulab: https://www.prekulab.com/

Promin: https://prominpku.com/overseas-ordering

Taranis Nutrition: https://www.taranis-nutrition.com/

Teva: https://www.tevapharm.com/teva-worldwide/

Vitaflo: https://www.nestlehealthscience.com/vitaflo

Resources

UK

Cambrooke: https://cambrooketherapeutics.co.uk/

Nutricia: https://www.nutricia.co.uk/patients-carers/living-with/low-protein-diet.html

ProminPKU: https://prominpku.com/ and https://prominpku.com/cake-ordering

Vitaflo: https://www.vitafriendspku.co.uk/

Fate Special Foods: https://www.fatespecialfoods.com/

Ireland

Nutricia: https://www.nutricia.ie/patients-carers/living-with/low-protein-diet.html

ProminPKU: http://prominpku.ie/

Vitaflo: https://www.vitafriendspku.co.uk/

US & Canada

Cambrooke: https://www.cambrooke.com/

Nutricia North America: https://nutricia-na.com

Australia and Aotearoa/New Zealand

Nutricia Australia: https://nutricia.com.au/ and https://lowproteinconnect.com.au/

Vitaflo Australia: https://www.nestlehealthscience.com.au/vitaflo/patient

Nutricia New Zealand: https://nutricia.co.nz/

Resources

Other names for PKU

PKU is short for Phenylketonuria, which was only discovered in the 1930s. Despite this short life in the scientific and medical world, it has been given various names.

Imbecillitas Phenylpyrouvica: This is the first name for PKU, and was used by Dr Følling following his discovery of the condition in 1934.

Oligophrenia Phenylpyruvica or Phenylpyruvic Pligophrenia: I have come across these two names for PKU, which use the same descriptors in reverse order. Both terms reference the presence of phenylpyruvic acid in the urine. As the news of the Dr Følling's discovery and simple diagnostic technique spread across the world, others began to look for PKU. Several published papers used these names instead of Følling's chosen name.

Følling's disease: This name for PKU is a direct nod to Dr Følling, who discovered the condition in 1934.

There were several other known inherited metabolic conditions in the first half of the 20th century, including alcaptonuria, pentosuria, and cystinuria. The names listed above were gradually phased out in favour of a new name, Phenylketonuria, which matched the nomenclature for these conditions. The name comes from the amino acid, phenylalanine, which is not correctly metabolised in those with PKU.

Hyperphenylalaninemia type 1: Hyperphenylalaninemia (HPA) is the name given to the condition of having too much phe in the blood. The 'type one' refers to the classic or severe type of PKU. There is on this classification in the chapter *Diagnosing PKU today*.

References

Part 1: What is PKU

Blau, N. (2016). 'Genetics of Phenylketonuria: Then and Now', Human Mutation: variation, informatics, and disease, 37(6), pp508-515. doi: https://doi.org/10.1002/humu.22980

Green, A. (2020). Sheila; unlocking the treatment for PKU. Redditch, UK: Brewin.

Hillert, A. et al. (2020). 'The Genetic Landscape and Epidemiology of Phenylketonuria', American Journal of Human Genetics, 107(2) pp 234-50. doi: https://doi.org/10.1016/j.ajhg.2020.06.006

Inwood, AC. et al. (2021). 'Australasian consensus guidelines for the management of phenylketonuria (PKU) throughout the lifespan' Human Genetics Society of Australasia Available at: https://www.hgsa.org.au/documents/item/8664 (Accessed February 2022).

MacDonald, A. (2021). Personal communication.

MacDonald, A, et al. (2020). 'PKU dietary handbook to accompany PKU guidelines' Orphanet Journal of Rare Diseases 15(171). doi: https://doi.org/10.1186/s13023-020-01391-y

Medscape (2017). Hyperphenylalaninemia. Available at https://emedicine.medscape.com/article/945180-overview (Accessed February 2022).

NHS website 1 (2022). Phenylketonuria. Available at https://www.nhs.uk/conditions/phenylketonuria/ (Accessed February 2022).

NPKUA (2022). Adults with PKU connection. Available at https://www.pku.com/about-pku/phe-in-the-brain (Accessed February 2022).

NPKUA (2014). PKU Medical guidelines. Available at https://www.npkua.org/What-is-PKU/PKU-Medical-Guidelines (Accessed February 2022).

NPKUA (2011). 'Chapter 2: Treatment and diet overview' PKU Binder. Available at https://www.npkua.org/What-is-PKU/My-PKU-Binder (Accessed February 2022).

O'Connor, P. (2020). Living with Mild Brain Injury: the difficulties of diagnosis and recovery from post-concussion syndrome. Abingdon, UK: Routledge.

SelfNutritionData (2018). Foods highest in Tyrosine Available at https://nutritiondata.self.com/foods-011087000000000000000-1.html (Accessed February 2022).

van Spronsen, F.J. et al. (2017). 'Key European guidelines for the diagnosis and management of patients with phenylketonuria', The Lancet 5(9) pp 743-56. doi: https://doi.org/10.1016/S2213-8587(16)30320-5.

Part 2: Why do we manage PKU

BBC News (2011). 'Brain changes seen in cabbies who take "The Knowledge"'BBC News, Health. Available at https://www.bbc.co.uk/news/health-16086233 (Accessed February 2022).

Brown, K.L. and Phillips, T.J. (2010). 'Nutrition and wound healing' Clinics in Dermatology 28(4) pp 432-439.doi: https://doi.org/10.1016/j.clindermatol.2010.03.028.

Bruinenberg, V. et al. (2017). 'Sleep Disturbances in Phenylketonuria: An Explorative Study in Men and Mice' Frontiers in Neurology 8(167). doi: 10.3389/fneur.2017.00167

Burlina, AP. et al. (2020). 'The Impact of a Slow-Release Large Neutral Amino Acids Supplement on Treatment Adherence in Adult Patients with Phenylketonuria' Nutrients 12(7) doi: 10.3390/nu12072078

Curtius, HC. et al. (1981) 'Serotonin and Dopamine Synthesis in Phenylketonuria.' Advances in Experimental Medicine and Biology, 133. doi:https://doi.org/10.1007/978-1-4684-3860-416

Farrell, DJ., and Bower, L. (2003) 'Fatal water intoxication'. Journal of Clinical Pathology 56 pp803-804. doi: http://dx.doi.org/10.1136/jcp.56.10.803-a

Ford, S. (2022). Personal communication.

Healy-Stoffel, M. and Levant, B. (2018) 'N-3(Omega-3) Fatty Acids: Effects on Brain Dopamine Systems and Potential Role in the Etiology and Treatment of Neuropsychiatric Disorders' CNS & Neurological Disorders – Drug Targets 17(3) pp216-232. doi: https://dx.doi.org/10.2174%2F1871527317666180412153612

Jenkins, TA. et al. (2016). 'Influence of Tryptophan and Serotonin on Mood and Cognition with a Possible Role of the Gut-Brain Axis' Nutrients 8(56). doi: https://dx.doi.org/10.3390%2Fnu8010056

Lamoreux, K. (2021). 'Serotonin Deficiency: What We Do and Don't Know' Healthline website. Available at https://www.healthline.com/health/serotonin-deficiency (Accessed February 2022).

Lienard, S. (2018). 'What is the dopamine diet?' BBC Good Food website https://www.bbcgoodfood.com/howto/guide/what-dopamine-diet (Accessed February 2022).

McGilchrist, S (2011). 'Music 'releases mood-enhancing chemical in the brain' BBC News website Available at https://

www.bbc.co.uk/news/health-12135590 (Accessed February 2022).

Nardecchiaa, F. et al. (2019). 'Clinical characterisation of tremor in patients with phenylketonuria' Molecular Genetics and Metabolism 128(1-2) pp 53-56. doi: https://doi.org/10.1016/j.ymgme.2019.05.017

Ney, D.M. et al. (2009). 'Nutritional management of PKU with glycomacropeptide from cheese whey.' Inherited Metabolic Disease, 32(1). doi:https://doi.org/10.1007/s10545-008-0952-4

NHS website 2 (2022). Overview - Selective serotonin reuptake inhibitors (SSRIs). Available at https://www.nhs.uk/mental-health/talking-therapies-medicine-treatments/medicines-and-psychiatry/ssri-antidepressants/overview/ (Accessed February 2022).

NHS website 3 (2022). Causes - Restless legs syndrome. Available at

https://www.nhs.uk/conditions/restless-legs-syndrome/causes/(Accessed February 2022).

O'Connor, P. (2020). Living with Mild Brain Injury: the difficulties of diagnosis and recovery from post-concussion syndrome. Abingdon, UK: Routledge.

Pérez–Dueñas, B. et al.(2005). 'Characterization of tremor in phenylketonuric patients.' Journal of Neurology 252 pp 1328–1334. doi: https://doi.org/10.1007/s00415-005-0860-6

Petzinger, G.M. et al. (2015) 'The Effects of Exercise on Dopamine Neurotransmission in Parkinson's Disease: Targeting Neuroplasticity to Modulate Basal Ganglia Circuitry'. Brain Plasticity 1(1) pp 29-30. DOI: 10.3233/BPL-150021.

Pietrangelo, A. (2019). 'How Does Dopamine Affect the Body?' Healthline website. Available at https://www.healthline.com/health/dopamine-effects (Accessed February 2022).

PKU.com website (2021). 'How PKU Affects the Brain' PKU.com, by BioMarin Available at https://www.pku.com/about-pku/phe-in-the-brain (Accessed February 2022).

Tompa, R. (2019) '5 unsolved mysteries about the brain' Neuroscience at the Allen Institute Available at https://alleninstitute.org/what-we-do/brain-science/news-press/articles/5-unsolved-mysteries-about-brain (Accessed February 2022).

Wollenberg, A. et al. (2018). 'Consensus-based European guidelines for treatment of atopic eczema (atopic dermatitis) in adults and children: part II' Journal of the European Academy of Dermatology and Venereology 32(6) pp 850-878. doi: https://doi.org/10.1111/jdv.14888

Part 3: How do we manage PKU?

Dietician's Life website (2015). 7 day 7 Exchange PKU Challenge Available athttps://www.dietitianslife.com/special-diets/the-7-day-7-exchange-pku-challenge/ (Accessed February 2022).

Ford, S., O'Driscoll, M., and MacDonald, A. (2018). 'Living with Phenylketonuria: Lessons from the PKU community' Molecular Genetics and Metabolism Reports 17 pp 57-63. Available at https://www.nspku.org/download/living-with-pku-lessons-from-the-pku-community/ (Accessed February 2022).

Green, A. (2020). Sheila; unlocking the treatment for PKU Redditch, UK: Brewin

Gregory, C., Yu, C., and Singh, R. (2007). 'Blood phenylalanine monitoring for dietary compliance among patients with phenylketonuria: comparison of methods.' Genetics in Medicine (9) pp 761–765. doi: https://doi.org/10.1097/GIM.0b013e318159a355

Jeong, JS., Kim, SK., and Park, SR. (2013). 'Amino acid analysis of dried blood spots for diagnosis of phenylketonuria using capillary electrophoresis-mass spectrometry equipped with a sheathless electrospray ionization interface' Analytical and Bioanalytical Chemistry (405) pp 8063–8072. doi:https://doi.org/10.1007/s00216-013-6999-6.

Koch, J.H. (1997). 'The PKU story' The Robert Guthrie Legacy Project Available at https://robertguthriepku.org/professional/ (Accessed February 2022).

MacDonald, A., et al. (2020) 'PKU dietary handbook to accompany PKU guidelines'. Orphanet Journal of Rare Diseases 15. DOI: https://doi.org/10.1186/s13023-020-01391-y

Mazzola, P.N., et al. (2015). 'Acute exercise in treated phenylketonuria patients: Physical activity and biochemical response' Molecular Genetics and Metabolism Reports 5, pp 55-9. doi: https://doi.org/10.1016/j.ymgmr.2015.10.003

Ney, D.M., et al. (2016). 'Glycomacropeptide for nutritional management of phenylketonuria: a randomized, controlled, crossover trial' The American Journal of Clinical Nutrition 104(2), pp334-345. doi: https://doi.org/10.3945/ajcn.116.135293

NPKUA, YouTube (2020). 'Virtual PKU Series: Home Phe Monitor Webinar' National PKU Alliance Available at https://www.youtube.com/watch?v=d9MnEcGqeGI(Accessed February 2022).
Salmons, E. (2016). 'Blood test advice' News and Views 152, pp18-19. Available at https://www.nspku.org/blood-test-advice/ (Accessed February 2022).

Stroup, BM. et al., (2016) 'Clinical relevance of the discrepancy in phenylalanine concentrations analyzed using tandem mass spectrometry compared with ion-exchange chromatography in phenylketonuria' Molecular Genetics and Metabolism Vol. 16, Issue 6, pages 21-6. DOI:10.1016/j.ymgmr.2016.01.001 Available at https://pubmed.ncbi.nlm.nih.gov/27014575/ Accessed February 2022.

van Wegberg, A.M.J., et al. (2017). 'The complete European guidelines on Phenylketonuria: diagnosis and treatment' Orphanet Journal of Rare Diseases 12(162). doi: https://doi.org/10.1016/j.ymgmr.2016.01.001

Wikipedia website (2022). 'SHS International' Wikipedia, the free encyclopaedia Available at https://en.wikipedia.org/wiki/SHS_International (Accessed February 2022).

Zaki, O.K., et al. (2016). 'The Use of Glycomacropeptide in Dietary Management of Phenylketonuria.' Journal of Nutrition and Metabolism doi:https://doi.org/10.1155/2016/2453027

Part 4: PKU and mental health

BBC Bitesized website (2022. Does willpower really exist? Available at https://www.bbc.co.uk/bitesize/articles/zk6spg8 (Accessed February 2022).

Bilder, D.A., et al. (2017). 'Neuropsychiatric comorbidities in adults with phenylketonuria: A retrospective cohort study.' Molecular Genetics and Metabolism 121(1) pp1-8. doi: https://doi.org/10.1016/j.ymgme.2017.03.002

Clacy, A., Sharman, R., and McGill, J. (2014). 'Depression, anxiety, and stress in young adults with phenylketonuria: associations with biochemistry.' Journal of Developmental & Behavioral Pediatrics 35(6) pp388-91. doi: https://doi.org/10.1097/dbp.0000000000000072

Cohunt, M. (2018). 'Choice overload: Why decision-making can be so hard' Medical News Today. Available at https://www.medicalnewstoday.com/articles/323243 (Accessed February 2022).

References & Bibliography

Ford, S., O'Driscoll, M., and MacDonald, A. (2018). 'Living with Phenylketonuria: Lessons from the PKU community' Molecular Genetics and Metabolism Reports 17 pp57-63. Available at https://www.nspku.org/download/living-with-pku-lessons-from-the-pku-community/ (Accessed February 2022).

McKeller, P. (2020) 'Suzanne Ford: Adults' Diet for life – lifelong PKU experiences. Mevalia UK.

NHS website (2022). Depression Available at https://www.nhs.uk/mental-health/conditions/depression/ (Accessed February 2022).

NHS website 2(2022). 10 medical reasons for feeling tired, Available at https://www.nhs.uk/live-well/sleep-and-tiredness/10-medical-reasons-for-feeling-tired/ (Accessed February 2022).

Oaklander, M. (2016). 'This Type of Food Makes You Feel Fuller Longer' Time website Available at https://time.com/4246736/protein-satiety-fullness/ (Accessed February 2022).

Reutskaja, E., et al. 'Choice overload reduces neural signatures of choice set value in dorsal striatum and anterior cingulate cortex.' Nature Human Behaviour' 2 pp925–935. doi: https://doi.org/10.1038/s41562-018-0440-2

Smith, L. (2020). 'Why lockdown is making us feel exhausted' Patient website UK. Available at https://patient.info/news-and-features/why-lockdown-is-making-us-feel-exhausted (Accessed February 2020).

StatsNZ website (2019). 'New Zealand's population reflects growing diversity' Stats NZ Tatauranga Aotearoa Available at https://www.stats.govt.nz/news/new-zealands-population-reflects-growing-diversity (Accessed February 2022).

Turland, A. (2021). 'Training the mind for better health' NSPKU News & Views 167, pp18-21. NSPKU: UK.

Part 5: Living with PKU

Adams, S. (n.d.). 'Protein Needs for the Athlete on a Low Protein Diet' Nutricia Low Protein Connect UK website Available at https://www.lowproteinconnect.com/Your-World/Protein-Needs-for-the-Athlete-on-a-Low-Protein-Diet-by-Sarah-Adams,-Senior-Metabolic-Dietitian/ (Accessed February 2022).

Buckland, K (n.d.). 'PKU & Fitness - The Challenge of Weight Loss' Nutricia Low Protein Connect UK Website Available at https://www.lowproteinconnect.com/Your-World/PKU---Fitness---The-Challenge-of-Weight-Loss/(Accessed February 2022).

Haas, D., et al. (2021). 'Differences of Phenylalanine Concentrations in Dried Blood Spots and in Plasma: Erythrocytes as a Neglected Component for This Observation' Metabolites 11(10). doi: 10.3390/metabo11100680

Holland, K. (2018). 'Menstruation: Facts, Statistics, and You' Healthline Website Available at https://www.healthline.com/health/facts-statistics-menstruation (Accessed February 2022).

MacLeod, E.L., & Ney, D.M. (2010). 'Nutritional Management of Phenylketonuria' Annales Nestlé (English ed.) 68(2). doi: https://doi.org/10.1159/000312813

NHS website 1 (n.d.). 'Limitations of BMI section of BMI healthy weight calculator' NHS website. Available at https://www.nhs.uk/live-well/healthy-weight/bmi-calculator/ (Accessed February 2022).

NHS website 2 (n.d.). 'Should you lose weight fast' NHS Available at https://www.nhs.uk/live-well/healthy-weight/should-you-lose-weight-fast/ (Accessed February 2022).

Robertson, L.V., et al. (2013). 'Body mass index in adult patients with diet-treated phenylketonuria' Journal of Human Nutrition and Dietetics 26(S1). doi: https://doi.org/10.1111/jhn.12054

Part 6: Beyond the restricted diet therapy

BioMarin (n.d.). 'PALYNZIQ® (pegvaliase-pqpz) Injection for PKU' BioMarin website Available at https://www.biomarin.com/products/palynziq/ (Accessed February 2022).

Gen website (2021). 'Engineered Bacterial Therapeutics Get Boost from PKU Study Data' Gen: Genetic Engineering & Biotechnology News Available at https://www.genengnews.com/news/engineered-bacterial-therapeutics-get-boost-from-pku-study-data/ (Accessed February 2022).

NSPKU (2017). 'Kuvan facts' NSPKU website Available at https://www.nspku.org/documents/?wpdmc=treatment (Accessed February 2022).

Bibliography

Criado Perez, C. (2019). Invisible Women: Exposing Data Bias in a World Designed for Men. London, UK: Vintage Books.

Følling, A., and Closs, K. (1938). 'Über das Vorkommen von 1-Phenylalanin in Harn und Blut bei Imbecillitas phenylpyrouvica.' 254(2) pp. 115-116. doi: https://doi.org/10.1515/bchm2.1938.254.2.115

Green, A. (2020). Sheila; unlocking the treatment for PKU, Redditch, UK: Brewin Books.

Messner, D.A. (2012). 'On the Scent: the discovery of PKU' Science History Institute: Distillations website https://www.sciencehistory.org/distillations/on-the-scent-the-discovery-of-pku (Accessed February 2022).

University of Cambridge (n.d.) MRC Cognition and Brain Sciences Unit at Cambridge University website. Available at: https://www.mrc-cbu.cam.ac.uk/ (Accessed February 2020).

NHS England (2018). Evidence review: Sapropterin for phenylketonuria. The NICE Medicines and Technologies Programme on behalf of NHS England Specialised Commissioning. Available at https://www.england.nhs.uk/(Accessed February 2022).

Schuett, V. (1994). 'The Discovery of PKU' National PKU News website. Available at https://pkunews.org/the-discovery-of-pku/ (Accessed February 2022).

University of Glasgow website, (n.d.). 'Forrester Cockburn' The University of Glasgow Story. Available at https://www.universitystory.gla.ac.uk/biography/?id=WH2187&type=P (Accessed February 2022).

van Spronsen, F.J., et al. (2017). 'Key European guidelines for the diagnosis and management of patients with phenylketonuria', The Lancet 5(9) pp743-56. doi: https://doi.org/10.1016/S2213-8587(16)30320-5.

Glossary

Amino acid A building block of protein. There are hundreds of amino acids which are put together in various forms to make different types of protein. Phenylalanine is an amino acid.

Anabolism The process by which the body builds muscle & tissue. May cause a small reduction in phenylalanine levels as protein is used to make new muscle & tissue.

Aspartame An artificial sweetener which contains phenylalanine, and which must be avoided by those with PKU. It may also be listed on food products as E951

Birmingham Children's Hospital A hospital in the city of Birmingham, UK. The restricted diet therapy for PKU was developed here in the early 1950s. It is still a centre for PKU treatment and research.

Blood/Brain barrier A tightly packed layer of cells which either prevents or allows different molecules to pass between the brain and the blood. Think of it as the brain's security system.

Blood phe level A measurement of the amount of phenylalanine present in someone's blood. Commonly determined using a blood spot.

Blood Spot A test to determine the levels of phenylalanine in a person's blood. This test involves dripping spots of blood onto an absorbent, medical card; hence the name. Also called a Guthrie test.

Catabolism The process by which the body starts to break down its tissues. This may be beneficial in losing excess weight, or harmful if too much phenylalanine is released back into the blood of someone with PKU.

Glossary

CBT see Cognitive Behavioural Therapy

Classical PKU The first type of PKU which was discovered in the 1930s, now refers to a severe form of PKU.

Cognitive Behavioural Therapy A type of talking therapy which may help to manage some health issues by changing the habits of behaviour and thought.

Dopamine A neurotransmitter assists with communication in the brain, commonly known as 'the reward hormone'.

E951 The additive number for aspartame. May be used in a list of ingredients instead of the word aspartame.

Enzyme A compound used in biology, and by the human body, to break down substances, including amino acids. Each amino acid is broken down by its own enzyme. Phenylalanine is broken down by phenylalanine hydroxylase.

Essential amino acid An amino acid which humans need, but cannot make themselves. They are usually sourced from food. Phenylalanine is an essential amino acid.

Guthrie test see Blood Spot

Glycomacropeptide A protein which is low in phenylalanine. In the early 21st century, it was developed for use in a new generation of PKU supplements. Often called GMP.

GMP see Glycomacropeptide

HPA see hyperphenylalaninemia

Hyperphenylalaninemia The condition of having too much phenylalanine in the blood, usually caused by PKU.

IEM see Inborn Error of Metabolism

IMD see Inherited Metabolic Disorder

Inborn Error of Metabolism A disorder in humans caused by the reduced or missing activity of an enzyme(s). Also known as an Inherited Metabolic Disorder.

Inherited Metabolic Disorder A disorder in humans caused by the reduced or missing activity of an enzyme(s). Also known as an Inborn Error of Metabolism.

Kuvan A brand name for sapropterin, used by BioMarin, a pharmaceutical company.

Large Neutral Amino Acids A group of amino acids which play a critical role in metabolism, commonly referred to as LNAAs. Phenylalanine is an LNAA.

LNAAs see Large Neutral Amino Acids

low-phe A food or drink which is considered low in phenylalanine. This term has various meanings due to differences in the severity of PKU. In this book, it refers to foods which have 2g of protein, or less.

Neurogenesis The process of a brain creating new neurons.

Neurons Specialised brain cells which transmit information.

Neuroplasticity The concept that the brain can change with training or learning.

Neurotransmitters Substances which neurons use for communication in the brain.

Mild PKU A type of PKU which still requires treatment, but where the patients are allowed a higher daily allowance of protein than those with Classical PKU.

PAH see Phenylalanine hydroxylase

Palynziq A brand name for PEG-PAL, used by BioMarin, a pharmaceutical company.

Glossary

PEG-PAL A new treatment developed in the 21st century which is administered as an injection.

phe see Phenylalanine

phe-free A food or drink which is considered to be free of phenylalanine for the purposes of a PKU restricted diet therapy.

Phenylalanine Often referred to as phe. An essential amino acid. People with PKU must restrict phenylalanine as they have restricted availability of the enzyme, phenylalanine hydroxylase, which breaks down phenylalanine. Often referred to as phe.

Phenylalanine hydroxylase The enzyme which breaks down the amino acid phenylalanine. Commonly referred to as PAH.

Phenylketonuria An Inherited Metabolic Disorder where the body cannot process phenylalanine.

PKU see Phenylketonuria

PKU restricted diet therapy A medical therapy where PKU is treated though the severe restriction of high-protein foods, and the administration of medical supplements.

Psyllium husks The phe-free husk of the psyllium plant. These husks are useful in the PKU restricted diet therapy, as they can improve the satiety and texture of baked goods & pancakes.

Restricted Diet Therapy The process of treating a medical condition though the restriction of food or drink. Not to be confused with a diet undertaken by choice.

Sapropterin A medicine in pill form, developed in the 21st century which may help 1 in 4 patients to manage their PKU.

Satiety The feeling of being full after eating.

Glossary

Serotonin A neurotransmitter which is used to communicate in the brain, and which may influence a person's mood, understanding, and memory functions.

Supplements An integral part of the PKU restricted diet therapy which provide amino acids and other nutrients which are not available through foods to those following the treatment. Often called 'medicine' or 'special drink'. Supplements are available in a wide variety of flavours and formats, including tablets.

Tyr see Tyrosine

Tyrosine An amino acid which humans need and which is usually sourced from the metabolism of phenylalanine. Because people with Phenylketonuria have an impaired metabolism of phenylalanine, they may need to source tyrosine from medical supplements. Tyrosine is included in most PKU supplements.

Index

acceptance 157

ageing 126

alcohol 214-215

amino acid: amino acid supplement see supplement; explanation of 19, 21-22; in foods 51; see also phenylalanine, tyrosine

anabolic 84-86, 229-230; see also exercise

anxiety 135-139

apps 180-181; see also habits, planning, routine

aspartame 48, 64, 118-119

baking 209-214; see also birthdays, psyllium husks

bbq 206-207; see also eating out

BH4 see sapropterin

Bickel, Dr 33-38

birthdays 207-211; see also baking

blood/brain barrier 23, 64, 233-234; see also large neutral amino acids

blood phe levels: 23-26, 75-80; factors affecting 81-86; for diagnosis 41-42; in non-PKU 41; recommendations & guideline for 42-43

blood spot test: 39-40, 75-78; at home 78-80

BMI 225-227; see also exercise

brain 57-62, 64-69; see also blood/brain barrier

breastfeeding 219

bullying 122-123

cakes 207-211; see also baking, celebrations

catabolic 81-83, 229-230; see also exercise

celebrations 205-215; see also eating out

Christmas 211-214

classical PKU 41

clinics: 87-94; changing 91-92; finding a clinic 254; making it work 89-91; see also food diaries

Cockburn, Prof. 44-45

community 159-163; benefits of 162-163

depression 155-158

diet for life 53-54

dopamine 24, 67-69; see also neurotransmitters, serotonin

E951 see aspartame

Index

eating in public: avoidance of 151-153; see also eating out

eating non-PKU food: 149-151; on holiday 196

eating out: 144-145, 187-193; email for 190-191; tips for 191-193; see also travel

Egeland, Borgny 27-31

emigrating 203-204; see also travel

emotional burden 134-170

enzyme 21-22; co-factor 236-237; replacement therapy 237-240; see also new treatments, PEG-PAL, phenylalanine hydroxylase

exercise 83-85, 227-230; see also healthy eating

exchanges 50-52;

fad diets 142-144

fatigue 156-158

financial assistance 120, 252

Følling's disease 30, 259

Følling, Dr 27-31, 259

food: and abnormal behaviours 147-153; commercial foods 116-120, 256-257; cost of 120, 252; see also specialised medical foods

food diaries 93-94, 179-181

gene therapy 242-245; see also new treatments

genetics of PKU 218-219

glycomacropeptide see GMP

GMP 107-110; see also supplements

growth: reduction in rate of 82; spurt/increase in rate of 84

gut absorption therapy 241 see also new treatments

Guthrie, Dr 39-40, 75-78

Guthrie test see blood spot test

habits 173-181

hanger / hangry 183-186

healthy eating 224-227 see also hanger, planning, satiety

holiday 195-202, and skipping diet 196; letters for 197-198

honesty with PKU 187

Hickman, Dr Evelyn 36

hunger 183-186

Hyperphenylalaninemia 41-42

IEM/inborn error of metabolism see inherited metabolic disorder

illness 83

injection see PEGPAL

imbecillitas phenylpyrouvica 29-30, 259

Index

IMD / inherited metabolic disorder 20-21

isolation, social 141-146

Jones, Mary 33-38

Jones, Sheila 33-38

Kuvan see sapropterin

large neutral amino acids 64, 233-234

LNAAs see large neutral amino acids

losing weight see weight loss

menstrual cycle 84, 219-222

mental health 127-170; how activity affects mood 160-165; see also acceptance, anxiety, depression, fatigue, spoon theory, vomiting

mild PKU 41-42

mindfulness 137-139

nappy test 39

neurogenesis 61

neuroplasticity 61-62

neurotransmitters 24, 64-69

new treatments 231-245

nights out see alcohol

oligophrenia phenylpyruvica 30, 259

orphan disorder 97

orphan drug 97

other treatments 231-245

PAH see phenylalanine hydroxylase

Palynziq see PEG-PAL

PEG-PAL 237-240

Pegvaliase see PEG-PAL

periods 84, 219-222

phe daily allowance 49-52; see also phenylalanine

phe-free food 51; lists of 256-257

phenylalanine: 19, 22, 30-31, ; metabolism of 21-22; toxicity of 63-71; see also amino acid, enzyme, tyrosine

phenylalanine hydroxylase 22; 236; see also enzyme, phenylalanine

Phenylketonuria: explanation of 19-26, diagnosis of 39-45; discovery of 27-38; incidence (how rare it is) 21, 218-219; inheritance (how it is passed on) 218-219; in the real world 187; new treatments for 231-245; returning to treatment 60-62, 253-254; types of 24, 41-42;

phenylpyruvic acid 28-31

PKU see Phenylketonuria

Index

PKU diet see restricted diet therapy

planning 173-181; see also habits, routine, travel

PPA see phenylpyruvic acid

pregnancy 84, 217-219

psyllium husks: 185: baking with 210

Quorn 48

recipes 146

restricted diet therapy 47-54; development of 33-38; for life 53-54; general rules 47-48; key components of 54; other treatments 231-245, returning to 60-62, 253-254; taking break 196; see also LNAAs, PEG-PAL, sapropterin

routine: 173-181; tips for 178-181 see also habits, planning

sapropterin 234-237

satiety 184-186; see also psyllium husks

serotonin 24, 65-67; see also dopamine, neurotransmitters

sleep and PKU 71, 155-158

sneaking food see eating non-PKU food

specialised medical foods: 115-116; delivery of 116; lists of 248-251, 257-258

spoon theory 158

Sunday roast 205-206 see also Christmas

supplements 53-54, 95-113; development of 33-38, 96-100; difficult flavour 36-37, 95-99; effects on blood phe levels 81-82; measuring dosage 99-102; remembering to take 112-113; travelling with 19-202; types of 102-104; see also GMP; why take them 64, 110-111

talking about PKU 167-170; FAQs 168-170

travel 195-204; clinic letters for 197-198; leaving diet for 196; supplements and 198

tyr see tyrosine

tyrosine: 22, 68-70; in skin repair 69-70; in supplements 67; see also amino acid, essential amino acid, phenylalanine

vomiting 148-149

weight loss 225-227 see also healthy eating, exercise

Woolfe, Dr 35

www.ingramcontent.com/pod-product-compliance
Lightning Source LLC
Chambersburg PA
CBHW070914030426
42336CB00014BA/2413